The Global Biopolitics of the IUD

The Global Biopolitics of the IUD

How Science Constructs Contraceptive Users and Women's Bodies

Chikako Takeshita

The MIT Press
Cambridge, Massachusetts
London, England

This book was set in Stone Sans and Stone Serif by Graphic Composition, Inc., Bogart, Georgia.

Library of Congress Cataloging-in-Publication Data

Takeshita, Chikako, 1963–
The global biopolitics of the IUD : how science constructs contraceptive users and women's bodies / Chikako Takeshita.
     p.   cm. — (Inside technology)
Includes bibliographical references and index.
ISBN 978-0-262-01658-2 (hardcover : alk. paper)
ISBN 978-0-262-54784-0 (paperback)
1. Intrauterine contraceptives. 2. Biopolitics. 3. Women—Health and hygiene—Political aspects. 4. Women—Health and hygiene—Social aspects. I. Title.
RG137.3.T35   2012
618.1'852—dc22

                                                                        2011010113

For my parents

Contents

Preface

Growing up in Japan, I was oblivious to the controversy around the intra-uterine device (IUD) that took place in the United States and elsewhere during the 1970s and 1980s. In fact, I had never even heard of IUDs until about a dozen years ago, after I moved to the United States. During an unrelated conversation, a prominent women's health activist and population studies scholar told me that scholars outside of international family planning had taken little notice of this contraceptive method despite its prevalence overseas. She believed that this was due in part to the device's damaged reputation in the United States. "But IUDs can help women control their fertility," she remarked, "particularly in pro-natal societies because women can use them secretly when their husbands object to contraception." Although I knew very little about the device, the complex history involving diverse women's lives behind this technology came through in her comments. This brief interaction left a strong impression on me, and I eventually launched the study that resulted in this book.[1]

This book investigates the development, marketing, and use of the IUD, tracing five decades (1960s to 2000s) of scientific activities and discourse surrounding the device. I have approached the subject from a feminist science and technology studies (STS) perspective, with the goal of illuminating the politics and processes of knowledge formation in contraceptive research that have had a significant impact on women's health and lives. I discovered in the writings of researchers, supporters, and opponents of the IUD how discursive relationships between contraceptive technologies and women's bodies were formed, re-formed, and multiplied over time. I engaged in the analytical work of tracing and accounting for the shifts in the scientific discourse while simultaneously investigating the broader historical, social, and political contexts within which IUD researchers were operating. Accounting for the past fifty years of the history of this technology in the United States and globally was like putting together a giant multidimensional puzzle that then had to be taken apart to compose separate chapters. This book offers a multifaceted picture of the historical roots of and the complex interactions among the heterogeneous constructions of this contraceptive device and its users.

Since I embarked on this project, I have had two IUD insertions. This was a way to embody my research subject, as well as an act of reproductive self-determination. I have explored the relationship between my personal and academic engagements with the device in a journal article, "The IUD in Me."[2] In this book, I occasionally weave my own encounters with the IUD into the analyses as examples of how an American user might experience the device today. Here, I disclose my satisfaction with this birth control method, not as a positive appreciation of the device, but to acknowledge the situatedness of my knowledge making. I am following a feminist research methodology that calls for anchoring objectivity in accounts of my own values, experiences, social positions, and relationship with my research subject.[3] This methodology made me aware of the fact that my embodied experiences are a product of my historical and geographical positionality, which directed me to attend to how different women's bodies marked by their race, class, and nationality are implicated by contraceptive research. In order to address the larger power relationships, this work constantly situates scientific discourses and technological objects within a complex transnational web of interests in reproduction, sexuality, and health.

Although I did not formally interview any women in my research, many people voluntarily shared with me their own experiences with the IUD. I learned that two of my friends had obtained the Dalkon Shield as young, emancipated women in the early 1970s and lost their ability to bear children as a result of severe infections brought on by the device. A colleague reminded me that IUD users today still experience significant health risks, although incidents of serious infections and uterine perforations are presumably rare. She recently spent an agonizing and painful few months when an IUD she received postpartum "got lost." Eventually found in her abdomen, the device required surgical removal. She swears she would never get an IUD again. Women also shared their favorable perspectives with me. A staff member at a campus women's center told me she was very disappointed when she could no longer get a replacement for her device after pharmaceutical companies withdrew IUD products from the American market in the mid-1980s. A friend shared with me that she had gotten pregnant after a heavy menstrual bleeding episode expelled her device without her knowledge. She completed her story by telling me that despite the mishap, she is using the IUD again because she feels that this contraceptive method best meets her needs. These personal exchanges served as a reminder that my critique of the device needs to reflect multiple perspectives. These diverse experiences are interlaced with the stories of technological development told in this book.

Personal stories of IUD users from the global South were harder to come by. I learned about them through texts written by anthropologists, reproductive health scholars, and women's health activists. Their stories convey a variety of relationships women have with the IUD in countries where the device is promoted through government-sponsored family planning programs and the challenges women face in seeking reproductive control are compounded by local gender dynamics. One episode that stood out for me was about a woman in rural Tajikistan who kept her husband from fetching a midwife and made him attend the birth of their fourth daughter himself. After witnessing the arduous childbirth, he gave up his desire to have a son and agreed to let his wife use an IUD.[4] The various ways in which women in Nigeria, China, Tajikistan, Uzbekistan, and Bangladesh have sought or resisted IUDs in attempts to take charge of their own reproductive health are discussed in my previously published article.[5] Although this book focuses on scientific activities and discourses around contraceptive technologies, I do not forget women's sometimes sobering and at other times heartening stories. In fact, by disentangling the backstories of contraceptive research, this book illuminates how social interests, political stakes, and cultural values have shaped and reshaped the ways in which reproductive choices for women are discursively and materially constructed.

Acknowledgments

I am indebted to many people whose intellectual and personal support made this book possible. I first recognize the Science and Technology Studies Graduate Program at Virginia Tech for fostering the interdisciplinary foundation of this work. Special thanks go to Tim Luke for mentoring me throughout my years there and to the present. My gratitude also goes to the Women's Studies Program at the University of California, Santa Barbara, for giving me an opportunity to focus on this project for a year. I am grateful to my colleagues in the Department of Women's Studies at the University of California, Riverside, for supporting my work and energizing me with their outstanding feminist scholarship. Being in their company deepened my commitment to integrate feminist theory into this book.

The research and writing for this book were financially supported by a grant from the Rockefeller Archive Center; the doctoral fellowship program hosted by the Women's Studies Program at the University of California, Santa Barbara; funding provided by Virginia Tech, the University of California, Riverside, and the University of California Regents; and the American Fellowship Summer/Short-Term Research Publication Grant awarded by the Association of American University Women. Archival research was assisted by librarians at the Rockefeller Archive Center in New York and the Sophia Smith Collection at Smith College in Northampton, Massachusetts.

I thank all those who read parts of the manuscript or attended my talks at various stages of this project and gave me invaluable feedback. They include Eileen Boris, Amalia Cabezas, Piya Chatterjee, Ben Cohen, Crissy Crockett, Gary Downey, Christine Gailey, Wyatt Galusky, Sherine Hafez, Bernice Hausman, Tammy Ho, Ann Laberge, Jane Lehr, Piyush Mathur, Martha McCaughey, Juliet McMullin, Jenifer Najera and the members of the dissertation fellow writing group, Laury Oaks, Jody Roberts, Christina

Schewenkel, Banu Subramaniam, Charis Thompson, Gerald Toal, and Margurite Waller. Saul Halfon was especially generous with his help on earlier iterations of this work. Thanks also to Jan Roselle for her careful reading and input on the manuscript at its final stage.

I am particularly grateful to Adele Clarke and Carole McCann for their extensive feedback. This book grew in depth and breadth thanks to their expertise and their insightful and generous advice.

My appreciation also goes to Marguerite Avery of the MIT Press, series editors of Inside Technology, and the rest of the editorial team. I thank as well the anonymous reviewers whose thoughtful comments greatly helped improve this book.

Finally, I thank my family, who made many sacrifices while I devoted a significant portion of my time and energy to this project. My parents have been unwaveringly supportive even though they have not been able to see their grandchildren as often as they would like. My daughters, Claire and Hana, brought me joy (as well as pain sometimes) and reminded me not to lose sight of the important things in life. And my heartfelt thanks go to Preston for his patience, love, and support.

1 Turning the Gaze on Modern Contraceptive Research: An Introduction

It has been a half-century since the contraceptive pill and the modern intrauterine device (IUD) were introduced. These inventions were remarkable because birth control methods before the 1960s had a number of drawbacks. Surgical sterilization prevented pregnancy with high reliability, but was invasive and not reversible. Barrier methods such as condoms, diaphragms, cervical caps, and sponges had high failure rates and required action at the time of sexual intercourse. The new contraceptives, prescribed by doctors, were coitus independent, were reversible, and had low pregnancy rates. At a time when abortion was illegal in the United States, these medical methods were saviors for women who dreaded unplanned pregnancies. Population control advocates, who sought to decrease fertility rates in the global South, also eagerly received these new contraceptives. They welcomed the IUD in particular as a one-time-intervention method that would prevent pregnancy for a number of years after the device was inserted.

In the past few decades, new birth control methods have been added. The female condom is a valuable addition to the barrier methods that simultaneously prevents sexually transmitted diseases (STD). Hormonal methods, which have been dominant, now include injections, implants, vaginal rings, patches, and the emergency contraception pill. The original oral contraceptive consisting of a high-dose combination of estrogen and progestin has been reformulated into safer lower-dose pills and progestin-only pills. Birth control pills that suppress menstruation are on the market as well. IUDs have been reformulated both materially and discursively, as this book discusses in detail. The "fit-them-and-forget-them" population control method has now become a "hassle-free contraceptive" for appreciative consumers. Research on male methods and contraceptive microbicides against HIV transmissions have also been underway, although their commercialization has been slow.[1] Despite these new products, women around the world still face impediments to safe and autonomous control of their reproduction.

Modern birth control technologies have simultaneously been a boon and a bane for women. Long-acting provider-controlled methods such as the IUD, injections, and implants are, as Adele Clarke labeled them, "imposable": they can be forced on women to contracept for a long period of time without allowing them to discontinue use at their own will.[2] Coercion in using these methods has been a serious violation of the autonomy of underprivileged women. Furthermore, all medical methods introduce the possibility of health impairment, which can range from minor physical discomfort to debilitating side effects, serious illnesses, and even threats to life. For many women, protection from pregnancy has come with a cost. Women in some societies who contracept against the wishes of their husbands or in-laws take considerable personal risks since angering them could lead to domestic violence and divorce. Without doubt, contraceptives have played an enormous role in enhancing women's lives by providing them with means to control their fertility. Yet medical contraceptives have also presented significant challenges to women's well-being.

Further complicating the significance of contraceptives, various groups—including the state, pharmaceutical industries, religious organizations, and feminist activists that are invested in the act of contraception for different ideological reasons—have assigned disparate meanings to this form of technological intervention in the body. For governments that regard overpopulation as a primary concern for the future of the state, contraceptives are the technological solution to a national problem. In economically developed regions where birth control is viewed as the responsibility or choice of the individual, government interventions are mostly limited to laws and policies guiding reproductive health care services. In these countries, the pharmaceutical industry and the market, social and religious values, and personal aspirations often have larger roles in shaping reproductive behaviors of their citizens. While curbing the birthrate of the poor and improving maternal health provide the framework for family planning in the global South, an entirely different set of concerns, such as profitability, liability, and health risks, determines the conditions of contraceptive use in the global North.

In both the global North and South, women's access to contraception undermines the traditional gender roles prized by religious conservatives and the political Right. These groups regard contraceptives as threatening technologies and actively try to discredit them as well as keep women from accessing them. Feminists have been struggling against the encroachment of antichoice movements on women's rights to reproductive freedom. Birth control technologies for women's health activists are a tool to enable women to take control of their reproductive destinies, although the technologies must be safe and used autonomously.

Contraceptive technologies are thus embedded in complex webs of state and nonstate investments in women's bodies, reproduction, health, and sexuality. This book begins from this assumption and examines how developers of modern IUDs have adapted to different social interests. It details how they understood the political stakes in women's bodies, justified their research activities, and presented their scientific findings in accordance with prevailing social norms. Prejudices against women of color and the lower classes, as well as assumptions about female sexuality, women's needs, and their behaviors, often guided scientific inquiries, reifying existing inequalities between women of the global North and South. While paying close attention to these biases, this book situates contraceptive research within broader transnational and racial political economies and shows that contraceptive development does much more than generate a technology that transforms the material body into a temporarily sterile organism. It argues that scientific work organizes itself in response to the socially and geographically diverse demands around fertility control and acts on women's bodies through its discourse.

At one level, this book uncovers how the IUD has manifested into what I call a *politically versatile technology*. Such a technology is adaptable to both feminist and nonfeminist reproductive politics, the result of the manifold efforts that its researchers undertook in order to maintain the suitability of the device as a contraceptive method for women in both the global South and North. New research and discursive rearrangements helped supporters of the IUD to neutralize criticisms against the coercibility of the device, respond to questions concerning its safety, counter opposition from the antiabortion movement, and turn the IUD into a marketable product as well as a popular family planning method. In other words, this politically versatile technology is a product of the discursive and scientific activities that took place around this contraceptive method over the past five decades. In this respect, this book is part of science and technology studies (STS) scholarship that "trace[s] the career of material things as they move through different settings and are attributed value."[3] In a sense, it is a biography of an artifact written through a feminist lens with an emphasis on the transformations of the scientific discourse over time and across geographies.

In another sense, this book is a theoretical exploration of the biopolitics of contraceptive research and development. It situates the scientific studies of a contraceptive method in what Michel Foucault called "biopower"—political interest in the regulation and governance of life, health, and the body in modern societies.[4] The network of biopolitical interests around fertility control and women's health has expanded over the past fifty years of IUD development with changing global political stakes, new social and market pressures, and scientific developments. IUD developers responded to these changes as they engaged new reasons and ways to regulate the female body with their invention. Their scientific discourse created profiles of potential users of varying races, classes, nationalities, ages, numbers of children, and presumed social conduct with various ideas about how women's bodies were best managed. This book shows how the manifold relationships between body and technology that we see among different IUD users were constructed and woven into the biopolitical network of the device, entwining reproductive lives of past and present, upper and lower class, young and old, religious and nonreligious, the global North and the South. In sum, we find a microcosm of the global political economy of women's bodies in the history of this contraceptive device.

Why a Book on the IUD?

As a seemingly mundane plastic object, the IUD has received scant attention from feminist STS scholars compared to oral contraceptives. Pills have provided an amalgam of topics to investigate, including the discovery of sex hormones, invention of synthetic steroids, the social forces and individual actors behind the development of the pill, the ethical implications of testing the method in Puerto Rico, and women's responses to the first highly effective scientific means of birth control. Nelly Oudshoorn's *Beyond the Natural Body* (1994) and Adele Clarke's *Disciplining Reproduction* (1998), for instance, are groundbreaking feminist STS works on these topics.[5] Yet studies focused on hormonal contraceptives have had relatively little to say about IUDs besides their role in population control and the disaster story of one form of IUD, the Dalkon Shield.

Among the variety of contraceptives, the IUD deserves scholarly attention. There are 150 million users around the world. It is the second most prevalent fertility control method in the global South, after female sterilization, and ranks fourth in the global North, after the pill, condoms, and female sterilization.[6] The 2010 Bill and Melinda Gates Foundation award that granted funding for an Indian researcher's innovation that aims to improve the copper-bearing IUD attests to the continued relevance of this contraceptive method to global reproductive health.[7] As the number of users continues to grow in the global South, IUDs are becoming more popular in the North as well. Positive images created through advertisements and good reception from a new generation of doctors are resulting in a proliferation of the device.[8] This contraceptive method will likely affect the reproductive lives of many more women in the years to come.

The recent acceptance of the IUD in the United States is in notable contrast to its earlier negative association with health risks, the medical community's neglect of women's well-being, and corporate greed, which became prominent concerns after many women were injured and a number of lawsuits drove pharmaceutical companies to withdraw their products from the American market during the mid-1980s. The new image of this contraceptive method as innocuous and liberating in its promotional materials is also difficult to reconcile with the role it sometimes plays as a coercive fertility control method in overzealous population policies and discriminatory practices against underprivileged women. Has the IUD been transformed from an oppressive and dangerous device to a niche consumer product? If so, how? This book shows that the ways in which women's bodies are subjected to this contraceptive method have not only changed but also multiplied over the years.

As an imposable contraceptive method, the IUD embodies the paradox of the simultaneous possibility of giving women control over their bodies and taking it away from them. Moreover, as a modern contraceptive with a long history of research and development, the device offers a unique opportunity to analyze how shifting political interests in women's bodies coalesced with the knowledge formation processes. STS and feminist scholars, however, have largely overlooked these significant analytical possibilities.

This book thus addresses the gap in feminist STS work on contraceptives as well as capitalizes on the richness of the IUD as an object of study to improve our understanding of the complex configurations of power and knowledge involved in scientific endeavors that manifest as women's unequal relationships with technoscience.

Feminist Perspectives on the IUD: A Review

When the IUD was introduced to American women in the mid-1960s, a few years after oral contraceptives had become widely available, women's health activists initially welcomed the device as an alternative birth control method. As doubts over the pill's safety began to rise in the late 1960s, women's health activists endorsed the IUD as a favorable method, including Barbara Seaman, whose influential 1969 book, *The Doctor's Case against the Pill*, led to the 1970 congressional hearings on the safety of the oral contraceptive.[9]

By the mid-1970s, the IUD faced its own controversy over health risks. Thousands of women wearing IUDs, the Dalkon Shield in particular, experienced infections, many of which resulted in septic abortions or permanent infertility, and at least fifteen died.[10] In her 1977 book, Seaman again discussed the IUD at length, this time in an explicitly cautionary tone.[11] Fueled by the class action lawsuit against the distributor of the Dalkon Shield in the 1980s, the IUD became a symbol of health disaster for women. During the 1990s, several feminist scholars published books on the Dalkon Shield that are highly critical of all IUDs and doctors, the pharmaceutical industry, and regulators that did not promptly and appropriately respond to women's complaints and disregarded the dangers of the device.[12]

Feminist scholars have also denounced the device's capacity for abuse. Analyzing the early activities around IUD development in the 1960s, Andrea Tone's 1999 article, "Violence by Design," criticizes population control advocates, who envisioned the device as a one-time insertion contraceptive method to be forced on passive female subjects, particularly the poor and uneducated masses. Using a patented device that punctures the womb in order to keep the device in place as an illustrative example, Tone argues that the IUD was a "technological violence inflicted against the female body."[13] Betsy Hartmann made a related critique in her 1995 book, *Reproductive Rights and Wrongs*, in which she condemns the overzealous attempt to control population growth at the expense of potential health risks to women. She points out that the IUD is a favored means of population control in a number of countries in the global South, where many women are given the device without consent, denied removal, and not properly informed of its health risks or treated for dangerous complications.[14] These feminist authors assert that IUD development was a masculinist project that disregarded women's well-being, and they portray the device as an inherently oppressive technology.

Some recent reproductive health activists of the global South offer a perspective that diverges from these negative viewpoints. During the United Nations Conference on Population and Development in Cairo in 1994, feminist activists managed to draw more attention to the importance of empowering women through broader social transformations in enabling them to exercise reproductive self-determination.[15] In the new discourse of women-centered family planning, which defines family planning as a basic right for women rather than a means for population control, an IUD is regarded as an option in the mix of contraceptive offerings that may meet the need of a woman. Ruth Dixon-Mueller, a prominent feminist scholar and international women's health activist, is among those who take such a position.[16] Gloria Feldt, former president of the Planned Parenthood Federation of America, also supports the IUD as one of the safe birth control methods that help women fulfill their rights, particularly in the face of the war on choice waged by the political Right and antiabortionists in the United States.[17] In contrast to the radical feminist perspective that regards the IUD as a problematic technology, Dixon-Mueller and Feldt deem the contraceptive inherently neutral. Instead of problematizing the device itself, they focus on the context of its use: improving access to all contraceptive methods, eliminating significant health risks, and protecting women's reproductive self-determination.

Local and global power relationships affect how well a woman is able to attain reproductive health and freedom. In line with Dixon-Mueller and other feminists who drafted the 1994 United Nations Cairo Consensus, I believe that women's social empowerment is a prerequisite to reproductive self-determination and well-being. However, I neither take the position that the IUD is fundamentally politically neutral nor believe it is intrinsically oppressive, as Tone and Hartmann imply. My view on technologies follows an STS perspective that artifacts become imbued with politics as they are constructed discursively as well as materially and as they are used in situated practices.[18] In this regard, feminist STS scholar Anni Dugdale's constructivist study is the precursor to my work. She argues that the metal Gräfenberg ring IUD was construed as an emancipatory tool for women during the 1920s in the context of the European sex reform movement and that plastic IUDs subsequently were reconfigured into a mass fertility control device in the context of the population control movement in the 1960s.[19] Her published work, however, ends with this period.[20]

Feminist scholarship on the IUD has thus been limited to critique of the device as a population control tool and analysis of the events around the Dalkon Shield. Even as the technology continued to develop in different directions, these works are frozen in time at a moment when the developers were most arrogant about their intent and overconfident about the device's ability to control women's bodies. This book extends into previously unanalyzed time frames and aspects of the IUD and the scientific activities around it.

Significantly, this book reinvigorates feminist studies of contraceptive research by integrating methodological insights from three overlapping yet distinct bodies of scholarship. First, it builds on STS scholarship that emphasizes the contextualization of scientific knowledge production and investigates the heterogeneous co-configuration of technology, users, and the body. Second, it develops an understanding of how gender, race, class, and nationality are factored into knowledge-making processes and how configurations of racialized gender are built into objects and practices. This approach is underpinned by antiracist and transnational feminist scholars' sustained attention to *intersectionality* or the understanding that women's access to power and experience of oppressions are not uniform because they are shaped by the subject's gender, race, nationality, and other intersecting categories. Finally, I rely on Foucault's notion of biopower to ground the complex network of problematizations and investments in the body within which lie the activities of contraceptive research. After providing a historical background to contextualize the start of modern IUD research, the rest of this chapter expands on these three analytical frameworks, concluding with an overview of the book.

Contextualizing IUD Development: A Historical Background

The changing landscape that created complex operational environments for contraceptive researchers of the past fifty years consisted of social movements, economic pressures, stricter regulations, transforming medical practices, the emergence of new technologies and scientific knowledge, and shifting norms around fertility control and cultural perceptions of menstruation. In the chapters that follow, I elucidate these elements as they arise and shape the context of scientific knowledge production of a particular kind. To set the stage for the rest of the book, I focus here on two fundamentals that remained stable and ran deep throughout the life cycle of IUD development despite the various transformations that occurred around it: the developers' inclinations toward neo-Malthusian ideology and the Population Council as their institutional progenitor and hub.

Neo-Malthusianism: The Ideological Core

The neo-Malthusian movement revived the ideas of the late-eighteenth-century British scholar Thomas Malthus, who predicted that overpopulation would cause famine, disease, and widespread mortality, and applied them to the contemporary economic situation. Mid-twentieth-century neo-Malthusians viewed "population increase as the main cause of poverty and correspondingly sought population reduction as a key economic intervention," particularly in the global South.[21] The population establishment began to coalesce around 1952 among philanthropists, scientists, and activists who were dedicated to the cause involving institutions such as the Population Council, International Planned Parenthood Federation, United Nations, and Ford and Rockefeller Foundations. The movement asserted an urgent need to avert a population explosion in the global South and that unless the birthrates in economically poor countries dropped, famine, economic collapse, environmental devastation, political turmoil, global instability, national conversions to communism, and even nuclear war were imminent.[22] Neo-Malthusianism's gained momentum is exemplified by Paul Ehrlich's 1968 bestseller, *The Population Bomb*, in which he urged the public to take action.[23]

The neo-Malthusian movement accommodated eugenics thinking that regarded the reproduction of certain groups of people as more valuable and worthy than others. The eugenics discourse that promoted improving the quality of the biological constitution of the population by selective breeding (or exterminating as the Nazis did) had won many followers during the interwar period.[24] When the eugenics movement lost its acceptance due to Nazi atrocities, those who supported eugenics causes adopted crypto-eugenics to maintain a low profile.[25] They thus pursued their goals without using the word *eugenics,* instead pushing it by other means, which often involved coalescing with, or being sheltered by, the neo-Malthusian movement. The strong identification between eugenicists and neo-Malthusians is demonstrated in the fact that six of the ten men on the Population Council's demographic and medical advisory boards had been associated with eugenics.[26] Consequently, as Linda Gordon, feminist historian of the birth and population control movements, points out, the "leading purveyors" of the anxiety about overpopulation "repeated on an international scale the motifs of eugenics sensibility, notably, the distinction between the moderate, restrained 'us' and the teeming, profligate 'them'."[27]

Hugh Davis, the inventor of the Dalkon Shield, exemplifies a neo-Malthusian who was also entrenched in eugenics. His eugenicist position is apparent from the explicitly racist and classist comment he made during the 1970 congressional hearings on the safety of the pill:

It is especially tragic that for the individual who needs birth control the most—the poor, the disadvantaged, and the ghetto-dwelling black—the oral contraceptives carry a particularly high hazard of pregnancy as compared with methods requiring less motivation. . . . It is the suburban middle-class woman who has become the chronic user of the oral contraceptives in the United States in the past decade, getting her prescription renewed month after month and year after year without missing a single tablet. Therein, in my opinion, lies the real hazard of the presently available oral contraceptives.[28]

Davis's neo-Malthusian conviction is expressed in his 1971 book promoting the IUD, in which he asserted, "We are losing the population war globally," and warned that the world would suffer global famine unless family planning were increased twenty-fold in the developing nations.[29]

Other neo-Malthusians masked their true beliefs with humanitarianism. William Vogt, director of the Planned Parenthood Federation of America, asserted that population control programs "can be sold on the basis of the mother's health and the health of other children. . . . There will be no trouble getting into foreign countries on that basis."[30] In other words, incorporating humanitarian aspects of birth control into the language of neo-Malthusians was a strategy to avert criticism and gain acceptance for intervening in the affairs of other nations.

The twentieth-century neo-Malthusian movement was populated by wealthy philanthropists, ideologues, nongovernment organizations such as the Population Council and the International Planned Parenthood Federation, and reproductive scientists who were joined by women's advocates like Margaret Sanger. Matthew Connelly shows that population-related advocacy groups that emerged after World War II had divergent roles and slightly different foci, which ranged from economic development and protecting the environment to women's well-being and cryptoeugenics. Decentralization made it easier for the movement to survive attacks and appeal to different constituencies. While seemingly diverse, the actors shared an ideology of modernity that upheld the small family and restrictive reproduction as the solution to poverty and economic development. Key leaders sat on multiple overlapping boards, which enabled them to "steer ostensibly independent organizations in the same direction."[31] Neo-Malthusiasm expanded most rapidly "where people of money and leisure took an interest and formed voluntary associations," making it a strongly upper-class-based activism.[32]

By the late 1960s, population control advocates managed to convince the World Health Organization (WHO) to take on family planning as one of its programs and establish the United Nations Population Fund (UNFPA). Meanwhile, regarding the intergovernmental organizations' capability as insufficient, neo-Malthusians continued to work together to pursue their cause. As these elite activists played key roles in convincing governments of the global South to back population limitation policies, the movement was practically driving neocolonialist projects. Initially fertility control was too controversial a terrain for the U.S. government and its Agency for International Development (USAID) to venture into. John F. Kennedy's administration simply urged private foundations to take the lead on the issue. Yet as the next president, Lyndon Johnson, became increasingly frustrated with having to provide aid to India in the form of food supplies, he started applying pressure on the country to take its population problem seriously.[33] By 1967, $35 million of the budget of the USAID was earmarked for family planning; during its peak between 1968 and 1972, U.S. government aid accounted for 80 percent of all international assistance for population programs. American foreign aid put such great emphasis on family planning during the late 1960s and 1970s that it shortchanged other types of aid. The head of the USAID population program, Reimert Ravenholt, "inundated" countries in the global South with free contraceptives, including IUDs, and abortion kits believing that flooding the region with birth control methods would lead to more acceptance and use. By 1979, the United States had paid for over 70 percent of the world's research in reproduction and contraception.[34] As the country gradually dominated international population programs and exerted its influence overseas in steering the global South toward fertility reduction, the neo-Malthusian movement increasingly became an imperialist project of the United States.

Overpopulation had been a geopolitical matter during the interwar period in Europe, when the redistribution of growing populations necessitated international agreements on migration and occupation of underexploited land and territory: the population problem was a matter of peace and war.[35] During the postwar years, overpopulation was reconceptualized in tune with the major conflict of the time: the cold war. U.S. leaders feared that poverty and overcrowding in developing countries would lead to political unrest and make them vulnerable to communist takeover, an apprehension that was amplified by the anxiety over the possibility of nuclear bomb attacks.[36] American interests in promoting family programs abroad thus served the country's interest in protecting friendly territory and contributing to national security. This became the basis of viewing population explosion as a geopolitical problem. The pill and the IUD became available when the concern over the "population bomb" was reaching its peak. In the overlapping discourse of the cold war and the "war on population," contraceptives came to be seen as a weapon to fight these battles.

Neo-Malthusians were often referred to as "population controllers" or "population control advocates" because of their emphasis on fertility restriction. The term *population control*, however, has come to have a negative connotation, implying coercion and Western domination, and neo-Malthusians now prefer alternative terminologies. Hodgson and Watkins point out that *population stabilization* is the preferred term among neo-Malthusians who attempt to exorcise all hint of coercion.[37] According to Barrett and Frank, the phrase "unmet need in family planning" has replaced the terminology of population control.[38] The rhetoric of the population establishment has shifted over time and currently accommodates the feminist language adopted in the 1994 Cairo Consensus, concealing the movement's historical connection to racist, classist, and imperialist ideologies. Yet the idea that global population growth must be curbed remains strong among those who have promoted research on the IUD. The neo-Malthusian connection to the contraceptive device can also be traced through the Population Council.

The Population Council: The Institutional Backbone of the IUD

The Population Council is the most significant institution behind the development and maintenance of the modern IUD. It funded research, assisted the distribution of the device, and sustained the acceptability of this contraceptive method through research interventions on the part of its affiliates. Although many IUDs other than the council's have been developed and some communist countries including China, the former Soviet Union, and Cuba adopted the contraceptive method on their own, this organization was most instrumental in the continued improvement of the IUD.[39] As later chapters elaborate, it assisted the development of the device as a birth control method for both the global North and the global South.

The Population Council was established in 1952 with gifts from John D. Rockefeller III, who had long participated in population enterprises that orchestrated various collaborations aiming at population control. The council's mission was to "stimulate, encourage, promote, conduct, and support significant activities in the broad field of population."[40] In comparison to the Planned Parenthood Federation of America, which tried to establish its support network by appealing broadly to the public and sometimes through drawing attention to controversial issues, the Population Council kept a low profile and maintained its organizational legitimacy by promoting itself as a scientific, politically neutral, nonpropagandistic organization. Simultaneously, it procured research funds from the elite, such as the Ford Foundation, and later the USAID.[41] Soon after its establishment Rockefeller and the council's executive vice president, Frank Osborn, started hosting biweekly lunches that brought together representatives from the International Planned Parenthood Federation, the United Nations, the Ford and Rockefeller foundations, and major pharmaceutical companies. In historian Matthew Connelly's words, the Population Council became "not only the world's preeminent institute for policy-oriented research in demography and contraception, but also a nexus for all the other major players in the field."[42]

Over the years, the Population Council provided significant technical assistance to the demographic and family planning programs in the global South. It offered fellowships to personnel from around the globe, who were then trained at the council or an affiliated organization before they returned to their home countries. As Suzanne Onorato points out, "Placement of influential population specialists in internationally-strategic locations allow[ed] for widespread distribution of population experts and easy access for the Population Council in foreign countries."[43] The council also provided direct assistance to the global South for the development of family planning programs. By 1963, its consultants had played key roles in designing some of the first major birth control programs in Taiwan, South Korea, Turkey, and Tunisia. In response to overwhelming requests, the organization created a technical assistance division in 1964 with support from the Ford Foundation, and over the following year, it expanded its programs to Thailand, the Philippines, Kenya, Honduras, Barbados, Morocco, and Iran.[44] The council often secured official invitations for advisory missions, which proposed state-sponsored family planning programs while promising aid to the foreign government. When a government signed on, it provided further evidence of broad support and acceptability of population control and justified the investment of further resources.[45]

During its initial years, the council's biomedical division was reluctant to tarnish its image as an elite scientific institution by becoming involved in the development of contraceptive products. It focused instead on supporting basic science by mainly awarding research grants for reproductive physiology and for pathways that might interfere with reproduction, hoping that these studies would eventually contribute to the invention of fertility regulation methods suitable for population control. It also supported research in immunology with the anticipation that it would lead to a vaccine against pregnancy that could be easily administered en masse.[46] All of these scientific investigations, however, were far from ready for clinical application.

It was against this background that the Population Council and Alan Guttmacher, former president of the International Planned Parenthood Federation, took an interest in intrauterine contraception when two favorable clinical experiences were reported from Israel and Japan in 1959.[47] The council and Guttmacher felt that the IUD held "great promise as cheap, simple, and highly effective contraceptive method."[48] The "impossability" of the method was no doubt attractive. According to Onorato, the first three presidents of the Population Council—John D. Rockefeller III, Frederick Osborn, and Frank Notestein—had for over a decade "emphasized emphatically, and often controversially, the importance of developing low user-responsible and less expensive contraceptive methods as the main objective towards the control of fertility."[49] The contraceptive vaccine was envisioned as the future "low user-responsible" method; but the IUD seemed more promising since this contraceptive already existed.

Its interest in the IUD prompted the Population Council to reverse its policy against getting actively involved in contraceptive development. It awarded its first two research grants in 1961 to physicians Jack Lippes and Lazar Margulies, who had invented some of the earliest IUD models made of flexible plastic and experimented with them on their patients. During the 1960s in particular, the council devoted considerable resources to the IUD through grants and research conducted in its own Bio-Medical Division.[50] It also orchestrated the 1963–1968 Cooperative Statistical Program (CSP), a long-term, large-scale, multilocation clinical study aimed at establishing the scientific legitimacy of the method in order to overcome the American medical community's skepticism toward IUDs. Beginning in 1962, the council sponsored five international conferences on the IUD, with its most recent one in 2005. It also brought together collaborating scientists from multiple countries to develop contraceptive technologies and founded the International Committee for Contraception Research, which later developed the hormone-releasing IUD, better known as the Mirena on the U.S. market today.[51]

The Population Council's enthusiasm for the IUD as a solution to overpopulation reached its height in the mid-1960s. Its investment in IUD research peaked at $500,000 in 1965, and at its second international conference in 1964, Bernard Berelson, then vice president of the council, declared, "This simple device can and will change the history of the world."[52] Within a couple of years, however, optimism around this contraceptive method had begun to wane, as had the council's funding. Nevertheless, it continued to invest in research on IUDs by developing the copper-bearing and hormone-releasing devices as well as to cultivate channels of distribution. More important, researchers affiliated with IUD development have consistently stepped in to conduct additional studies and support the device's reputation whenever controversies arose that might weaken its status. Behind the stories I tell in the chapters that follow was a community of IUD researchers, many of them affiliated with the Population Council, who played the role of stewards of this contraceptive method.

The Co-Configuration of Technologies, Users, and Bodies

One of the analytical frameworks central to this book draws on the STS approach to the co-configuration of technology, users, and the body. Here I elaborate on how the focus on users enabled feminist STS scholars to address women in their studies of technologies.

Contraceptive research generally proceeded without the participation of women. Adele Clarke and Theresa Montini introduced the term *implicated actors* to draw attention to prospective users of contraceptives for whom the actions taken by researchers will be consequential.[53] More often than not, the implicated actors of contraceptive research have not been able to provide input, even though their profiles and characteristics as target recipients of the technology were imagined and discursively constructed by developers to legitimize their inventions. Investigating implicated users of contraceptives has been important to feminist scholars who seek to overcome the invisibility of women and include the analysis of power in their study of relationships between developers and users.[54]

The study of implicated actors has shed light on how contraceptive researchers garner support for their studies by suggesting potential users, how scientists organize their work around who they think the users are going to be, and how scientific activities are shaped by cultural values and social interests. Nelly Oudshoorn, for example, shows that rhetorical profiles of potential male users, such as the "caring and responsible man" and the "daring" man who exhibits bravery by trying out a new technology, has given researchers assurance that male contraceptive methods have viable prospective users. She observes that representations of users "can function as tools in enhancing the cultural feasibility of technology."[55] Jessika van Kammen's study of immunological contraceptives similarly illustrates that imagined users helped developers of the contraceptive vaccine anticipate the use of the technology.[56] These studies indicate that contraceptive researchers view their work as an effort to develop an appropriate solution for a particular set of women (or men) and organize their scientific work accordingly. They show how the scientific discourse coconstructs contraceptive technologies and their implicated users.

Anni Dugdale's work suggests that developers of the Gräfenberg ring and plastic IUDs also gained acceptance for their endeavors by aligning their technological inventions into popular social movements and representing their users accordingly. By casting his intrauterine ring as a new scientific contraceptive and a player in the sexual liberation movement of the early twentieth century, Ernst Gräfenberg presented his device as suitable for emancipated European women and their liberated bodies. Three decades later, neo-Malthusian developers promoted the "population-control" IUD while concurrently bolstering the idea that women of the global South were "overreproducing" and that their fertile bodies needed to be restrained.[57] I concur with Dugdale's argument that "technologies do not simply act on pre-given bodies, but bodies, technologies and subjects are made together, each being implicated in the production of the other."[58]

Attending to the semiotic meanings that are built around particular users is an analytical approach put forth by Steve Woolgar. As he argues, user configuration "define[s] the identity of putative users and set[s] constraints upon their likely future actions."[59] For instance, population control advocates' characterization of IUD users as women who will be made to accept fertility restriction measures imposed on them implied that their ability to take control of their own bodies would be significantly constrained. Designer-user relations, however, are not simply one-way streets: users as well as the objects themselves may play an active role in deinscribing or reinscribing meanings. As Madeleine Akrich argues, "We have to go back and forth continually between the designer and the user, between the designer's projected users and the real users, between the world inscribed in the object and the world described by its displacement."[60] Christina Lindsay also found in her study of computer users that "co-construction of users, user representations, and technology was not a static, one-time exercise by the designers . . . but was a dynamic ongoing process through the whole life history of the technology."[61] This book will similarly show that although IUD designers initially designated the device to be a coercible contraceptive method, they constantly had to adjust to the actual users and the different realities that the device encountered, and consequently had to reconfigure the technology along with its users and target bodies. In this sense, there were continuous reciprocal relationships among the designers, the object, and the subjects.

Examining this feedback loop, Dutch and Norwegian feminists have studied how technological innovations required a renegotiation of gender relations and an articulation and performance of gender identities.[62] Nelly Oudshoorn's study of male contraceptive development, for instance, shows that representations of contraceptive users had to reformulate cultural expectations around gender and that the rearticulation of gender identities was a crucial aspect of technological innovation. She reveals that in order to construct a male user who was compatible with manliness, developers had to rewrite cultural scripts of masculinity. Because dominant gender norms excluded men from taking responsibility for contraception, a new *gender script* that defines "caring" and "daring" men as manly had to be written into the male pill for it to be culturally acceptable.[63]

IUD development started with a gender script that rendered women passive recipients of contraceptive technologies. But along the way, developers also took into consideration the cultural significance of women's other identities (such as race, class, and nationality) and categories (such as marital status, age, and childbearing experience) and rearticulated subject identities whenever former representations of the device and its users became insufficient or no longer relevant or accepted. This feedback loop led to the generation of multiple *biopolitical scripts* for the IUD comprised of various co-configurations of the device, users, and the body.[64] As later chapters detail, the IUD came to embody multiple scenarios concerning diverse women, which resulted in the political versatility of this device. To uncover the transnational and domestic social inequities that are perpetuated in some of these scripts, we now turn to the theoretical frameworks that antiracist feminist theorists cultivated.

Diffraction as a Metaphor for Critical Feminist Consciousness

Diverse contraceptive users of different races, classes, and nationalities occupy disparate positions of power, while their reproductive capacities, health, and choices have historically been inequitably (de)valued. The eugenics and population control movements are clear examples of privileging the fertility of white upper- and middle-class women while attempting to undermine the reproductive capacities of women of color, lower classes, and the global South. Today, global capitalism provides the context for privileging the reproductive lives of those who have economic resources over those who do not. It is important to note that underprivileged women living in advanced capitalist countries have constituted a global South within the North.

Feminist scholars of color have pointed out that gender analyses that assume "women" as a universal category silence the experiences of women who are positioned disparately due to race, class, nationality, sexual orientation, and other factors that separate them from the normative white middle-class female Western citizen. They call for the problematization of interlocking systems of power and oppression through intersectional analyses that locate gender in its complex histories of race, class, sexuality, nationality, colonialism, imperialism, militarism, and other mechanisms of social stratification.[65] A feminist study of contraceptive research must take into account the power relations that affect women unequally within the processes of knowledge formation. This study thus examines how racist, classist, and Eurocentric ideas intersected with gender ideologies and directly and indirectly affected the course of contraceptive development.

Simultaneously this study offers a critique of how contraceptive researchers effortlessly erased presumed differences among women and depoliticize research activities by assuming that biology and technology are universal and that scientific knowledge claims apply to all women, whom they view as fundamentally similar physiologically. In order to discern the ways in which multiple research trajectories involving diverse implicated actors culminate in a seemingly singular object, I propose to use the *diffraction* metaphor. A theoretical term suggested by Donna Haraway and used by feminist scholars, diffraction as metaphor urges us not simply to reflect but to plot and plan for change.[66] My application of the concept stays close to the optical phenomenon of light waves bending as they pass through a prism and registering as multiple colors from which the singular light was made. As Haraway maintains, diffraction is a way of "seeing the history of how something came to 'be' as well as what it is simultaneously."[67]

If we take the commercialized state of the IUD as the unbroken light, diffracting it allows us to view the multiple developmental trajectories of this device. The fractured light rays represent how the IUD came to be, or the various meanings and developmental moments that are embodied by the final artifact. As Haraway suggests, to diffract an object means to reveal its historical passages, making it impossible for the artifact to hold a single meaning. Diffracting the IUD shows that it is not reducible to one thing because it is an amalgamation or assemblage of the different ways in which the scientific discourse appropriated women and control over their bodies. I am applying the diffraction metaphor to the history of technology in order to write a nonlinear, heterogeneous biography of this artifact.

In addition to enabling explicit historicization of a seemingly ahistorical object, diffraction as optical metaphor also makes visible the differences among women, which the scientific discourse effaces by reducing women's relationship with technology to female biology. The unbroken light represents the IUD as a neutral technology that has similar effects on all women who are biologically analogous. When the light is broken up and the multiple rays are exposed, these beams represent the diverse political interests in women's bodies that developers took into account as they engaged in scientific activities and produced authoritative knowledges. As Karen Barad explains, diffraction "makes light's wavelike behavior explicit."[68] It discerns how diverging reproductive politics intersected and how one technology became the catalyst for mitigating differences among women. It helps illuminate how the reproductive lives and contraceptive choices of women in the global North and South were, and continue to be, intertwined.

Diffraction can also be a metaphor for seeing things in different light. The effect of diffraction (or interference of light waves) is responsible for the way the hue of the iridescent colors on peacock feathers changes with the changing viewing position of the observer. Different light-reflecting angles also create the changing appearances on holographic stickers. Just as altered light interferences produce different color hues, textures, and images, different social positions, viewpoints, and situatedness significantly change the meanings that an object carries.

As a critical metaphor, diffraction offers a new "apparatus of investigation" into the "nature of difference" and "entanglement."[69] In this book, diffractive methodology illuminates the dynamics whereby IUD researchers simultaneously construct and obscure differences among women, as well as concurrently appropriate and efface women's agency. Furthermore, diffracting cultivates multiple feminist consciousnesses by enabling us to capture the complex interactions, interdependencies, and contradictions among the pursuits to control and enhance the reproductive lives of diverse women.

Contraceptive Research and Biopower

I now turn to the concept of biopower as an instrument to explore how contraceptive research and development are embedded in a web of interests in controlling populations and women's bodies. *Biopower* is a term coined by Michel Foucault, who observed that as modern societies developed, regulating life and bodies became central to their effective functioning.[70] Surveying the history of European modernization, he identified the emergence of two complementary techniques of power: one, concerned with the individual body as an organism, aims to "keep the body under surveillance, train it, use it, and if needed punish it," while the other deals with the population as a whole and attempts to affect life and bodies collectively.[71] Foucault named the technique of power that intervenes in individual bodies *disciplinary power,* which "secures its hold . . . by creating desires, attaching individuals to specific identities, and establishing norms against which individuals are judged and against which they police themselves."[72] He argued that biopolitics, or the technique of power that targets aggregate phenomena including the rate of reproduction and overall health of the population as political problems, extends its influence by creating statistical knowledge, forecasting trends, and implementing policies. Foucault theorized that by conjoining biopolitics and disciplinary power, emerging biopower allowed the modern state to gain control over life both collectively as population and individually as discrete bodies.

In *The History of Sexuality*, in which he introduced these concepts, Foucault identifies birth control (or the "Malthusian couple," as he characterized it) as one of the privileged objects of knowledge and an important technology of power that provides analytical access to both the individual body and the collective population as targets of control.[73] He also conceptualized medicine as the power-knowledge nexus that can be applied to both an individual organism and general biological processes. In other words, birth control and medicine as biopower have both disciplinary and regulatory effects.[74] Contraceptive research, then, can be understood as power-knowledge that partakes in biopower linking the bipolar ends. In other words, medical technologies resulting from contraceptive development physically control individual fertile bodies. Meanwhile, research produces knowledge concerning fertility control, which allows actions to be

taken on the population as a simultaneously scientific and political problem. Foucault's insights concerning the bipolar nature of biopower inform
my investigation of how strategies to act on collective lives are conjoined
with disciplinary mechanisms over the individual body.

Originally Foucault developed the concept of biopower in relation to
powers of the state. Upon recognizing the heterogeneity of institutional
forms invested in managing the population, he augmented the concept
by coining the term *governmentality*. This encompasses "a whole variety of
ways of problematizing and acting on individual and collective conduct
in the name of certain objectives which do not have the State as their
origin or point of reference."[75] Contraception is aptly conceptualized as
a form of governance because it is of interest not only to the state, but
also to individuals, medical professionals, religious authorities, and feminist activists. What constitutes an appropriate intervention in the female
body not only reflects national interests but is also shaped by the market, as well as cultural norms around gender, sexuality, and family. Furthermore, in advanced industrial societies, the norms of reproduction
are generated through individualism, medicalization, and consumerism.
In these societies, biopower is exercised through rendering fertility management as a responsibility of the individual to be enacted under medical
auspices and the consumption of medical products rather than an obligation to the state. Yet individual women are not the only ones with interests in the female body and its procreative capacities. Various agents
are invested in women's health, sexuality, abortion, and gender and class
relations. Consequently disciplinary mechanisms around contraception
are dispersed, taking heterogeneous forms such as state propaganda, pervasive cultural and religious norms, social policies, the medicalization of
reproductive lives, and advertisements that cultivate individual aspirations. Rather than considering biopower strictly in the sense of the bipolar structure of state power over population and individual bodies, my
work incorporates the state within the concept of governmentality. I will
refer to the diverse, diffused, and persistent forces over women's bodies as
modes of governance that are generated in conjunction with contraceptive
technologies.

The remainder of this section elaborates on the relevance of biopower
to this book. First, I characterize the neo-Malthusian movement, capitalism, patriarchy, and women's movements as globalized biopower in order

to situate contraceptive research among intricate webs of multiple global interests. Second, I compare this book to existing feminist scholarship that uses a Foucauldian approach to examine contraceptive technologies. Finally, I introduce the concepts of biopolitical subject and biopolitical script to facilitate the analysis of how the scientific discourse co-configures technologies, users, and governance over users' bodies.

Globalized Biopowers

Historians of demography have traditionally framed population control as a quintessential nation-building biopolitical governmentality, where the state is invested in shaping the quality, quantity, and mobility of the population.[76] My attention to global biopower does not override the importance of state-based biopolitical strategies that further the neo-Malthusian cause. Many states in the global South have employed some form of population policy as a project for building the nation-state, often echoing the idea that fertility reduction is "integral to modernization, enhancing the health and productivity of both poor people and poor countries."[77] Nation-based population programs such as those in India, Taiwan, and Korea served as platforms for testing IUD acceptance, and the outcomes had important implications for the future of the device.[78] China stands out as one nation that deployed the IUD widely as a biopolitical tool to limit the nation's population growth.[79] Vietnam followed suit during the late 1980s, instituting its own population policy modeled on China's one-child policy and heavy reliance on the IUD.[80]

Recently, however, scholars of population movements have begun to analyze the various mobilizations around population issues as transnational movements rather than on a nation-by-nation basis.[81] During the mid-twentieth century, neo-Malthusianism in particular transformed into a global biopolitical enterprise concerned with world population and with building its own version of modernity transnationally. It was a movement that did not necessarily have the state at its center, but operated through dispersed actors, including philanthropists, scientists, government agencies, and non- and intergovernmental organizations that "created a network of public and private agencies that constituted a novel form of global governance."[82] Contraceptive research promised to offer population controllers knowledge to regulate reproductive biology and medical products to control fertile bodies. In other words, neo-Malthusianism operated through both national and transnational biopowers, and contraceptive research produced technologies of global biopower.

Neo-Malthusianism is only one of the globalized biopowers that influenced the transformation of the IUD over time. Capitalism is another global engine that generates biopower. In advanced liberal capitalism, fertile bodies are of importance not only as sites of reproduction but also as agents of production and consumption. The pursuit of health, economic productivity, and happiness operates as the rationale behind technological interventions in the body at both population and individual levels. As global capitalism expands, technologically managed bodies serve not only national interests but markets beyond the national borders.

Patriarchy, or male dominance, is another kind of transnational biopower invested in controlling women's bodies. As Jana Sawicki notes, although Foucault intended to locate the processes through which women's bodies were controlled through discourses and practices of biopower, he never followed through on this.[83] Thus it has been left to feminist scholars to investigate biopower over women's bodies. Sandra Bartky's seminal article on disciplinary power illustrates how patriarchal power is expressed through the female body, which is disciplined into docile, ornamental, passive, unthreatening, and sexual being.[84] Sawicki draws attention to new reproductive technologies, suggesting that "if biopower was an indispensible element in the development of capitalism insofar as it made possible a controlled insertion of bodies into the machinery of production, then it must also have been indispensable to patriarchal power insofar as it provided instruments for the insertion of women's bodies into the machinery of reproduction."[85] This statement holds true in the context of many societies where fertility is a masculinity issue as much as it is an economic factor and where women have struggled for reproductive freedom.

Feminist historian Carole McCann makes explicit connections between patriarchy and the elite-led movements to curb global population growth.[86] She demonstrates that mid-twentieth-century neo-Malthusian demographic theory used racialized and imperialist (heteronormative) gender logics to organize its narrative. In other words, demographers assumed that the global South should follow traditional Western domestic arrangements as the ideal reproductive model and a marker of modernity. Simultaneously, the ideal model upheld the paternal figure of a man who supports his family while taking the initiative to keep it small. As such, patriarchal gender relations were readily embedded in the global neo-Malthusian movement that underpinned modern contraceptive development.

The antiabortion movement, as Rosalind Petchesky points out, is also inextricable from patriarchy.[87] During the 1980s, the political Right and religious conservatives in the United States gained their foothold by using the "pro-life" banner while pushing for the restoration of traditional patriarchal family structures that restrict sexual activities to married heterosexual couples.[88] Their biopolitical activities included advocating a multitude of policies that have a negative impact on women's control over their fertility and sexuality, including abstinence-only sex education, restrictions on foreign aid, and domestic health care reforms that constrain access to abortion and birth control information and services. Their disciplinary techniques include relentless campaigns aimed at talking women out of obtaining abortions and humiliating those who choose to end pregnancies. They have global alliances such as the Catholic church, which has long institutionalized globalized patriarchal biopower.

Feminists are concerned with making sure women have control over their bodies. While their organizations practice both locally and transnationally, the ideological commitment to improving women's social, economic, and health statuses is global. Thus neo-Malthusianism, capitalism, patriarchy, and feminism are all invested in women's bodies, while they coexist within the global economy, sometimes in conflict with and at other times in alliance with one another. Contraceptive technologies enable some and jeopardize other biopolitical agendas. Investigating how the IUD has been developed, challenged, and modified will illuminate how a complex and changing network of biopolitical interests has been woven around this device for over half a century.

Feminism, Biopower, and Disciplinary Technologies

Before examining the biopolitics of contraceptive research, a brief review of feminist readings of biopower and contraceptive technology is warranted. Departing from the earlier tendencies of feminist scholars to "reduc[e] all of Western medical science and technology to another example of violence against women,"[89] Jana Sawicki considers how "disciplinary technologies control the body through techniques that simultaneously render it more useful, more powerful, and more docile."[90] Adele Clarke aptly captures how birth control technologies do this to individual bodies: "Contraceptives are what Foucault termed 'disciplinary technologies,' part of the 'socialization of reproductive behavior' that can discipline such behavior in multiple ways. But, simultaneously, contraceptives can be means of liberation, offering strategies of resistance against related disciplines of gender as well as race, class, and global position."[91] In other words, contraceptive technologies are often introduced to women in combination with expectations about how to manage their fertility—spacing or limiting births, for instance; but women can also use contraceptives to benefit their lives and negotiate reproductive self-determination with their husbands or partners and the state.

This is indeed the case with IUDs. The device has been an agent of the state in many countries that seek to limit population growth, where IUD insertions have become normalized as an appropriate and expected reproductive behavior. Yet women have not always acquiesced to being the docile body of the Malthusian couple. As a reversible method, the IUD has offered women a window of resistance. As Susan Greenhalgh reports, village women in China who were required to wear an IUD after the birth of their first child often claimed to have lost their devices and conceived additional children beyond their permitted quota. For decades, Chinese IUDs were ring shaped and did not have a string protruding to the vagina, making them tamper resistant or more difficult to locate and remove. Although none of these women admitted that they had their IUD illegally extracted, Greenhalgh infers from the fact that many of these women had a daughter and then quickly became pregnant with their second child that they took physical and legal risks to get rid of their devices to conceive a son.[92] This is an example in which women resisted state intervention in their reproductive decision making by reversing the technology of governance.

In a pronatal society, a woman whose husband opposes contraception may use an IUD to control her fertility surreptitiously. Women's strategic use of the device to achieve reproductive self-determination has been reported from various parts of the world. Nancy Stark has observed that women in rural Bangladesh negotiated control over their fertility by secretly obtaining an IUD and later confessing to their husbands what they had done. She explains that the confession neutralizes the husband's anger and saves face for him, for he would be able to claim that he neither approved nor knew of his wife's contraception.[93] Monika Krengel and Katarian Greifeld illustrate how midwives in Uzbekistan act as official reproductive gatekeepers for the state, mandating who is allowed to become pregnant in accordance with the national population policy and each woman's reproductive profile. Uzbek midwives sometimes become allies of women who are pressured by their families to have more children than they desire. Quoting a midwife, the authors write: "It is a big relief for the woman when we say 'sit down, I shall insert an IUD for you.' The husband will not know about it. For a good purpose, one can also deceive."[94] Here, the goal of the state to limit births and a woman's desire to control her fertility converge using the same means: the IUD. This is an example in which a disciplinary technology simultaneously liberates women while it subjects them to a biopolitical intervention.

Tine Gammeltoft's extensive ethnographic work on Vietnamese women and IUDs also demonstrates how women experience and appropriate biopower.[95] Vietnamese women are subjected to pervasive state propaganda for small families, and health care workers constantly attempt to persuade village women to use contraception. The IUD is the preferred method of the state's family planning programs. The device's side effects of heavy bleeding and cramping, however, significantly compromise the health of village women. Yet while resenting their physical weakness, which they associate with IUD use, women also use it as an excuse to take a break from hard labor. Furthermore, women regard their ability to tolerate an IUD as fortunate since they are now less prone to frequent pregnancies, which they have come to view as unfavorable for their health and their family's economic well-being. Hence, although the IUD subjugates Vietnamese women to state biopolitics, this disciplinary power has also opened up possibilities for women to escape other hardships and create new subjectivities as IUD users.

These diverse workings of the IUD as a disciplinary technology echo feminist scholars' engagements with Foucauldian theory, which highlights resistance as copresent with power. Foucault held that power has more than a mechanical effect on subjects; it can change course at the site and be thwarted. In other words, on the one hand, the body is subjected to the disciplinary power of the IUD. Yet on the other hand, the body can turn itself into a productive, useful, and powerful entity by appropriating or resisting the technology. As Judith Butler's reading of Foucault suggests, "The body in subjection becomes the occasion and condition of productivity, where the latter is not finally separable from the former."[96] By virtue of having the body as an instrument, women gain certain possibilities for resistance and redirection of power. Feminist scholars' focus on Foucault's disciplinary power is understandable due to its theoretical possibilities for making resistance visible and changing the vector of power.

Reading accounts of regional IUD users through a feminist Foucauldian lens shows how disciplinary power over individual women's bodies simultaneously subjects them and opens up possibilities for empowerment. They demonstrate that whatever intentions IUD developers had, they did not produce any sort of absolute power. This book builds on these understandings but then departs from the dominant feminist approach that focuses on the downstream effect of biopower on individuals and their strategies of resistance. It investigates instead how contraceptive research generated governing forces over collective women's bodies upstream while keeping in sight the downstream implications on disciplinary powers over individual bodies.

Biopolitical Scripts of a Contraceptive Technology

This book follows the constructions of what I call the *biopolitical scripts* of the IUD, which involve three-way co-configurations of technologies, users, and modes of governance over the body. An exemplary biopolitical script of the IUD is that of the "population," which consists of constructions of a low-user-failure contraceptive technology, excessively fertile masses, and governing apparatuses that are geared toward reducing overall fertility rates through population policies, propaganda for small families, and health services that focus on birth control delivery. On the downstream, disciplinary power operates through family planning programs and normalization of contraceptive behavior—if not outright coercive and semicoercive insertions. A number of biopolitical scripts for individuals of economically advantaged groups are also identified as the book traces the development of the IUD. Generally, reproductive behaviors of "individuals" are governed by generating a desire to practice personal choice over parenting, lifestyle, and health.

It is worth pointing out here that there are two ways to think about "choice" as a biopolitical script. Paul Rabinow and Nikolas Rose point out that claims to a "right" to one's body, to health, and need emerged as a pushback against the instrumentalization of life as a political object.[97] Political struggles that seek to gain control over one's own body have long been fought by feminists in the birth control movement led by Margaret Sanger, the second wave feminist movement during the 1960s and 1970s, the transnational women's health movement of the 1994 United Nations meeting in Cairo, and beyond. One way to view women-initiated contraceptive choice is as a kind of resistance against biopower. Yet another way to view this rhetoric of rights is as another form of governance. Scholars of governmentality have indicated that "liberal subjects," or the citizens of liberal capitalist societies, are being ruled through freedom.[98] The normalized desire to maintain health and control one's life and body through the use of medical products guides individuals to take reproductive responsibility. The biopolitical script of a free society consists of the "practice of self," or self-governance, facilitated by the discourse of choice.[99]

This book details the multiple ways in which the IUD is constructed as a technological solution to a range of problems surrounding reproduction, health, and women's empowerment by teasing out the multiple biopolitical scripts it embodies. Simultaneously it illuminates how "differences" among women are built into the device and how diverse women are subjected to varied, diffused, and persistent powers over the body as biopolitical subjects of a medical technology.[100] Importantly, the rhetoric that supports IUD use in family planning is increasingly turning to the kinds of argument used in relation to the liberal subjects or the market and consumers, blurring the boundaries between collective and individual biopolitical subjects. By examining the ways in which various biopolitical scripts became integrated into contraceptive research, the chapters that follow show how different modes of governance over women's bodies are connected to one another, sometimes sustaining each other's logic and sometimes refuting it.

Notes on Methodology

I used a wide variety of sources for this book, ranging from scientific reports and material from the archives of the Population Council and Planned Parenthood to historical studies of reproductive politics. I consulted the proceedings of five international conferences on the IUD starting in 1962 and observed the last one in 2005 in person.[101] The earlier conference proceedings were particularly valuable in understanding the developers' thoughts on this contraceptive method and its users since they included transcripts of frank discussions among meeting participants. The *Population Reports*

on the IUD, which were published seven times between 1973 and 2005 by
the Johns Hopkins School of Public Health, were especially informative in
learning how the status of the device was represented to family planning
programs in the global South at particular times.[102] I parsed the mainstream
perspective presented in the Population Reports by consulting numerous
medical journal articles used to compile the report and analyzed how original studies were interpreted to formulate the official expert summary.

The annual reports of the Population Council, as well as the letters and
memoranda from the archives of the council and the Planned Parenthood
Federation, helped me understand some of the discussions that went on
behind the scenes of scientific activities.[103] An informal interview with a
key council population scientist and a thorough reading of his autobiog-
raphy provided me with an insider's perspective.[104] Monographs on the
Dalkon Shield were a valuable source of information for this device.[105] Anni
Dugdale's excellent dissertation on the social construction of the IUD from
1908 to 1988 contributed to my understanding of the device's history.[106]

As I investigated the scientific documents, I mapped the scientific activities against a wide range of social, cultural, and political backgrounds
in order to contextualize IUD development. Historical analyses of birth
control, population control, and the antiabortion movements, as well as
discussions of the 1994 Cairo Consensus, were important in understanding
the range of social movements within which the device holds importance.
I also took into account the developments of other contraceptives, such as
the pill, Norplant, and Depo-Provera, as context-setting factors for IUD research.[107] I read a number of reports from the field on IUD implementation
in family planning programs, as well as ethnographic accounts of women's
responses to this particular contraceptive method, all of which broadened
my understanding of its impact on women's lives.[108] Although I did not use
interviews as a formal method, personal conversations with women who
have or have had an IUD helped keep various experiences and perspectives
in mind.

Organization of the Book

The chapters roughly reflect the chronological development of research
on the IUD. Chapter 2 focuses on the first decade of its development, the
1960s. Chapters 3 and 4 span the first forty years on separate topics, and

chapter 5 takes the story to the present. Each chapter centers around a particular scientific interest. Chapter 2 shows that researchers were focused on improving and measuring the contraceptive efficacy of the device in the early phase of the development. Chapter 3 illustrates how researchers negotiated the safety of the IUD. Chapter 4 concerns the mechanism by which pregnancy is prevented as it relates to antiabortion politics. Finally chapter 5 highlights how side effects of a hormone-releasing IUD created a unique product. Each chapter examines the relationship between scientific activities and biopolitical interests, highlighting how different ways of conceptualizing the technology were coproduced with representations of diverse users and forms of governance. Chapters 2 through 4 also provide additional background for the discussion in chapter 5 concerning the development of the latest commercial IUD product, Mirena. Each chapter diffracts the IUD as a contraceptive method in different ways. Combined, the following four chapters provide a comprehensive picture of the heterogeneous construction of this contraceptive method.

More specifically, chapter 2 illustrates how the IUD was formulated as a technoscientific biopower, or a technological solution to what was widely viewed as a population problem. Two major scientific activities were conducted during the 1960s: the search for an ideal physical configuration of a device that would achieve a continuous occupation of the uterus and the large-scale clinical trial that successfully scientized this contraceptive method. The chapter analyzes IUD developers' efforts while critiquing the neocolonial agenda that underlay their scientific activities. As birth control for a nation rather than for an individual, the IUD was co-constructed with a representation of overfertile "masses" and assembly-line-style insertions in the global South as the preferred form of governance. This rather technocratic conceptualization of the contraceptive method did not last long but nevertheless became foundational to the device's existence.

Chapter 3 follows the IUD on the American market from its introduction in the mid-1960s to the early 2000s and examines how biopolitical subjects implicated by IUD development expanded from the masses to individuals. Controversy over IUD safety, which started in the early 1970s and continued into the mid-1980s, served as the pivot around which a series of scientific work investigating the health risks of the IUD emerged. The effort to rehabilitate the IUD as a safe technology entailed the construction of a "safe" user, namely, a monogamous mother. Continued marketing of the device to the American market as a birth control method for mothers also helped maintain the legitimacy of the device as a family planning method in the global South. The chapter illustrates how the production of biopolitical subjects involved considerations of a woman's race, class, geographical location, age, marital status, the number of children she already had, and anticipated social and sexual conducts.

Chapter 4 follows the scientific debate over the IUD's mechanism of action and investigates the alliance between contraceptive researchers and reproductive-choice feminists around this issue. Religious leaders and antichoice physicians argue that women have the right to choose not to use an IUD since it prevents pregnancy after fertilization. IUD supporters refute such characterization, maintaining instead that the device works primarily by preventing fertilization. The former claims to be speaking out on behalf of religious women, whereas the latter criticize their opponent as politically motivated. This ongoing struggle over scientific knowledge in the battle to win control over women's bodies represents the constitution of science as a power-knowledge nexus. The chapter also traces how neo-Malthusian contraceptive developers gradually adopted the feminist discourse of women's well-being in order to support their cause, while what is known as the "war on choice" strengthened the partnership between traditional contraceptive researchers and pro-choice feminists on both domestic and international fronts.

Chapter 5 shows how multiple research trajectories of the past are connected to current representations of the hormone-releasing IUD, Mirena, now blossoming as a commercial product in the United States. The chapter follows how this device came about through an independent historical trajectory because of its distinctive side effect: the dramatic reduction of menstrual bleeding. Deconstructing Mirena's promotional material, the chapter demonstrates how the biopolitics of the IUD evolved from a negative eugenics and population control device aimed at restraining the fertility of underprivileged, nonwhite, and global South populations to a positive eugenics method used to maintain the reproductive capacity of white upper-middle-class women in the global North. In addition, it has become a consumer product for women who seek a lifestyle free of menstrual periods. The story of Mirena reinforces the argument that the diversity of biopolitical subjects implicated in IUD research microcosmically reflects the transnational and racial political economies of women's bodies.

2 "Birth Control for a Nation": The IUD as Technoscientific Biopower

At the first international conference on the intrauterine device sponsored by the Population Council in 1962 in New York City, conference chairman Alan Guttmacher articulated the need for a new kind of contraceptive for what he referred to as the "masses": "The reason the restraint of population growth in these areas is moving so slowly is the fact that the methods we offer are Western methods, methods poorly suited to [non-Western] culture[s] and to the control of mass population growth. Our methods are largely birth control for the individual, not for a nation."[1]

Guttmacher, who was the chief of obstetrics and gynecology at Mount Sinai Hospital in New York City and would soon become the president of the Planned Parenthood Federation of America and a leader in the International Planned Parenthood Federation, implied that the available nonsurgical birth control methods at the time, such as barrier methods and the newly developed oral contraceptives, were suitable only for Westerners, who were presumed to be educated and motivated enough to use them correctly and consistently. By implicitly distinguishing Western individuals from non-Western users, he suggested that women in developing countries could not be trusted to use existing contraceptives. Simultaneously, he positioned the IUD as "birth control for a nation" and characterized its intended users as a disindividualized "mass" equated to a national "population."[2]

Guttmacher later described with fascination in his 1969 book *Birth Control and Love* how devices were inserted like machine parts into submissive women on an IUD installment assembly line in Hong Kong:

The best IUD manipulator I have observed was in Hong Kong. . . . Her record was seventy-five insertions in three hours[,] . . . that is one every two minutes and twenty-four seconds. Dr. Wong kept three nurses busy helping her. One was supervising the removal of panties of the next patient, the second nurse soothed the brow of the patient on the table and the third passed instruments to Dr. Wong. I have never seen such graceful hands, such exquisite economy of finger movement; there wasn't a false motion.[3]

Rather than considering fertility control as a complex social practice involving individuals, families, communities, and the state, his technocentric vision for reducing population size privileged the consecutive insertions of a device in machine-like bodies. Feminist scholars have criticized his remarks, aptly calling it "gynecological Taylorism."[4] Here I draw attention to the particular kind of power over the body that Guttmacher and his fellow IUD developers found desirable: a technoscientific biopower that is wielded using scientific knowledge making and technological solution.[5]

IUD enthusiasts during the 1960s shared the vision that population management was a matter of figuring out how best to manipulate the biological function of reproduction. It fell on some initial researchers to build what amounted to a machine part that efficiently controls the uterus. They used their skills and positions as scientists and physicians to test various devices to find out which one worked best in women. They also systematically measured how different models performed and produced authoritative studies about this contraceptive method. This chapter charts how women in the IUD discourse were stripped of agency as they were represented as "the population," reduced to the anatomy of their uteruses in scientific studies of the device, and converted into statistical data in clinical trials.

The scientific discourse and activities analyzed in this chapter took place during the 1960s and early 1970s. I start, however, by outlining the historical relationships among contraceptive development, population science, and Western imperialism. Drawing this connection enables us to see modern contraceptive research as an extension of colonial relationships and as a biopolitical endeavor enmeshed with the neo-Malthusian movement and the cold war. The main sections analyze the scientific activities aimed at perfecting and validating the modern IUD as a biopolitical tool. Researchers' focus on uterine physiology removed agency from users and relocated it to biology, making it more palatable for technological intervention without consideration of individual women's desires and conditions. Quantification of contraceptive performances had a similar effect of collapsing social differences into biological sameness. Altogether the analyses in this chapter illustrate how technoscientific biopower, or the will to intervene in life collectively using technological and scientific apparatuses, became the dominant framework for IUD development. Finally, I discuss how the technocratic vision of solving what some saw as the world's population problem began to falter toward the end of the 1960s as developers recognized that fertility reduction needed to be addressed as political and sociocultural issues rather than a technical one. I conclude that imposability nonetheless became strongly imprinted in the IUD during its first decade and became the foundation for other biopolitical scripts configured for the device later.

Science, Neocolonialism, and the War against Population

Science and Western Imperialism
A clear analysis of the rise and characteristics of IUD research needs to consider the co-constitutive relationship between science and Western imperialism that gave rise to population and reproductive sciences. During the eighteenth and nineteenth centuries, sciences—including biology, medicine, taxonomy, botany, geology, and geography—assisted and benefited from colonial projects in ways that we may describe as co-constitutive. European state ambitions to learn about, occupy, and reap profits from foreign lands were often assisted by science. Simultaneously, scientific activities gained justification from the mandate to accumulate knowledge about exotic organisms, peoples, and places. Colonial science, in short, allowed Europeans to classify, domesticate, own, and intervene in foreign places and the lives of their inhabitants.[6]

Nature and women's bodies became targets of domestication by colonial science. Feminist scholars such as Carolyn Merchant and Londa Schiebinger have argued that since the scientific revolution, science has viewed earth or nature as female—a territory to be explored, exploited, and controlled.[7] As Anne Fausto-Sterling effectively demonstrates in her study of nineteenth-century European scientists who dissected Sarah Bartmann (also known as the "hottentot Venus"), colonial scientific scrutiny over the "savage" African woman's body was an act of domination over colonial subjects and territories.[8] After probing, categorizing, and exposing the native woman's body, they proclaimed the biological inferiority of the colonial subject, which was used as scientific support for claims of European superiority and justification for colonial expansion and governance over the land of her origin. Fausto-Sterling also analyzes how the display of open sexuality and unfeminine behavior on the part of Sarah Bartmann provoked anxiety in the European scientists, for whom an untamed woman of color symbolically destabilized white male superiority in both their home country and abroad.[9]

The relationship between science and Western imperialism was twofold. First, advancements in science and territorial invasion had a codependent relationship since each legitimized the other. Second, scientific knowledge of colonial subjects and their homeland provided colonizers with discursive and practical tools for ensuring their continued domination. This centrality of science to Western expansion continued beyond the colonial era. The post–World War II modernization agenda for the Third World, orchestrated in conjunction with the establishment of the World Bank and the institutionalization of international development, depended on and at the same time it helped to advance the academic disciplines of economics, demography, and agriculture.[10] An interdependent relationship between scientific development and the maintenance of the Western world order was established whereby new theories of economics produced knowledge about "underdeveloped" countries measured by capitalist standards. This in turn gave authority to the World Bank and the International Monetary Fund to intervene with loans and aid for development projects that often had the effect of disrupting the local subsistence economy in the interest of fostering modernity. Economics thus became the power-knowledge nexus that provided the West with instruments to rule over the global South based on capitalist principles.

Demography was another genre of science that drew its legitimacy from promoting the Western world order while it created knowledge aimed at facilitating the Westernization of the rest of the world. When the study of population emerged as a scientific discipline around the 1920s and 1930s in the United States, demographers established themselves as a highly mathematical field, hoping that the implied objectivity of quantification would help dissociate them from political activists who were promoting birth control, eugenics, and immigration restriction. Despite its pretense to be apolitical, the field relied on government funding to do demographic work, and thus it developed close ties to U.S. foreign policy needs in the cold war era. Consequently the discipline became inevitably affiliated with the "preoccupation of U.S. population policy makers and their demographic advisers [to promote] family planning programs as virtually the only solution to the third-world population problem."[11] As Susan Greenhalgh, an anthropologist and scholar of population science, points out, demographic theories embraced modernist concerns based on underlying assumptions about Western supremacy. Population science presumed that fertility reduction is "caused by and in turn causes Westernization and that reproductive Westernization is good for everyone," because, its adherents believed, "Europe and its offshoots are superior to the rest of the world and the source of all significant change."[12] Demography became a "science that colonizes."[13]

Carole McCann traces the imperialist logic of mid-twentieth-century demography back to the original writings of Thomas Malthus and identifies the racialized gender logic that held together both the early Malthusian and the cold war population narratives.[14] Malthus's writing reflected the patriarchal imperial landscape of the late eighteenth century as he catalogued indigenous reproductive practices. He deemed their high fertility rates to be a sign of primitivism, as well as the cause of indigenous societies' savagery and extreme hardships, including famine. Malthus judged their gender relationships to be primitive and in contrast to those of the bourgeois, which he presented as the marker of modernity. McCann argues that twentieth-century demographers drew more than mathematics from Malthus's text, namely, the idea that the Western patriarchal family produced superior demographic results. Malthus's contemporary followers not only obtained "an authoritative map of the world" but also "reconfigured [it] for the demands of mid-twentieth century neocolonial masculine modernity."[15] Neo-Malthusian demographers adopted the idea that the small family and fertility management practices, adopted and implemented by economically rational and exemplary Western men through their wives' bodies, represented the normative gender relationship. Restrained reproductive behavior led by the man also signified competencies for a modern and a better life. As eugenics became unpopular after World War II, differences in reproductive practices filled in as the proxy for racial differences in defining hierarchical relationships among groups of people, especially between the global North and the South. As McCann illustrates, the gendered and colonial logics ran deep in mid-twentieth-century demographic theories. Reproductive science soon inherited these logics from population science, and neo-Malthusian thinking offered justification and legitimacy for contraceptive development.

Contraceptive Development and the War on Population

As Adele Clarke points out in her account of the history of reproductive science, early-twentieth-century reproductive scientists were "mavericks" in light of how birth control was a taboo topic and studying it was looked down on in the scientific community.[16] Reproductive scientists, like population scientists, tried to distance themselves from the political movements of birth control and population control. Yet they too "depended on them since these movements provided increasing support and legitimacy for reproductive research."[17] Reciprocally, the population control movement relied on scientific activities for the technological instruments to implement fertility regulation. This codependency between Western imperialism and scientific development applied to the IUD as well as the pill. Because the pill came first, it set the context for the emergence of the IUD.

Before the arrival of the pill, diaphragms combined with spermicides were considered the most reliable female-controlled contraceptive. Margaret Sanger, the most prominent leader of the early birth control movement in the United States, started advocating the diaphragm in 1915 as a method that "gave women a measure of self-determination in their reproductive lives" rather than leave them at the mercy of their male partners to use condoms or practice withdrawal.[18] Yet she became increasingly dissatisfied with this method by the late 1940s because of its limited utility for many women who lacked the sanitary conditions required to use a diaphragm hygienically. More important, women did not like this method because it required intimate physical contact (women had to use their hands to insert the diaphragm inside their vagina) and because of the inconvenience of having to follow a strict regime (each time before sex, diaphragms had to be applied with spermicide and inserted; they then had to be removed after a certain number of hours and cleaned).[19] The oral contraceptive, in contrast, was a coitus-independent method that avoided the "fuss and mess" of diaphragms altogether. When the pill was introduced in 1960 American women of all classes received the method's contraceptive reliability and the spontaneity it allowed with great enthusiasm, so much so that the pill became synonymous with the sexual revolution.[20]

The pill responded to both women's desire for "something better" and eugenicists' and population control advocates' interests. But the latter motivation was the primary force behind its development at its inception. During the early years of her birth control movement, Margaret Sanger made strong claims about women's rights over reproductive control and female sexual pleasure. However, as a pragmatic activist, she eventually dropped her radical rhetoric and cooperated with the eugenics and neo-Malthusian constituencies in order to gain cultural acceptance toward birth control practices.[21] By the time Sanger hired Gregory Pincus to develop the contraceptive pill in 1951 with money donated by millionaire birth control activist Katharine McCormick, she had become a population controller herself.[22] According to Linda Gordon, "[Sanger] believed there was an over-population crisis, that it was impoverishing much of the world's population, and that it represented dangerous opportunities for communism."[23] By then she had also come to believe that the diaphragm, which required individual fitting by doctors and proper insertion into the vagina each time a woman had intercourse, was not going to work in the global South. Disappointed in the diaphragm, Sanger aspired to create a "universal contraceptive" that would reliably limit the fertility of the poor, especially those in underdeveloped regions.[24] While sponsoring the research on hormonal contraception, she expressed her deep faith in "modern science," saying that it "ought to be able to [solve the problem]."[25]

Codependency between Western imperialism and science was solidified when Pincus and his collaborators decided to test the pill in Puerto Rico. After conducting some preliminary testing on American women, the researchers ran into legal restrictions in the United States that made it impossible to conduct clinical trials of contraceptives on a large scale. In 1956 they moved their study to the former U.S. colony, where interventions in Puerto Rican women's bodies and sexuality—from regulating prostitution to conducting sterilization campaigns—had been central to the American imperial enterprise since the nineteenth century.[26] The island, which had been regarded as having an overpopulation problem and subjected to multiple sterilization campaigns since the early twentieth century, also provided what Katharine McCormick called a "cage of ovulating females" necessary to carry out clinical tests.[27] Many of the Puerto Rican women in the pill trial experienced intolerable side effects such as severe headaches, bloating, and nausea that led them to drop out of the trial. As a result the local chief investigator concluded that the oral contraceptive could not be a universally acceptable drug.[28] Nevertheless, the clinical trials enabled the pill developers to collect the necessary data to obtain approval for the hormonal compound as a drug to treat menstrual disorders from the U.S. Food and Drug Administration (FDA) in 1957.[29] Scientific activity and imperialist intervention became integral to testing the pill; the knowledge-producing effort was combined with the regulation of the reproductive capacity of former colonial subjects.

Pincus's hormonal compound was approved as the first oral contraceptive by the FDA in 1960 at the height of the cold war when anxieties about communist expansion and nuclear war were at their apex. Advocates of population control in this context gave another meaning to the pill: ammunition against global unrest caused by overpopulation.[30] Senator Bob Dole's statement during the 1970 U.S. congressional hearings over the safety of the contraceptive pill exemplifies such sentiment. He warned against scaring women away from the drug, arguing that it was an "important weapon in the struggle to achieve some control over our ability to multiply ourselves into chaos."[31]

Market release of the pill set the stage for the revival of the IUD as a contraceptive method. When IUDs were introduced to American women in the early 1960s, they were readily viewed as a contraceptive that might better meet women's needs. Meanwhile, IUD developers, who regarded the pill as too user dependent to be effective in a concerted effort to limit births, were far more concerned with the prospect of developing a better weapon with which to fight the so-called war on population.

The Geopolitical and Biopolitical Missions of IUD Researchers

In his opening speech to the second international conference on the IUD in 1964, sponsored by the Population Council, John D. Rockefeller III evoked geopolitical and biopolitical apprehensions by declaring that the outlook for stemming the tremendous growth in world population appeared bleaker than the hope of preventing nuclear weapon use.[32] He then charged conference participants with a mission of using science to help avert population overgrowth and help maintain the world order:

In this effort, bio-medical scientists like yourselves have an important role to play. Your knowledge and wisdom can help guide and direct governmental policies and programs, your research findings will contribute significantly toward providing modern methodology for family limitation. Your work can thus be a major factor in the success of national family planning programs, upon which rest the hopes of many countries for economic survival and for the well-being of their people. . . . This meeting can be of historic importance in applying the knowledge from modern science to a major world problem to the great benefit of human kind.[33]

His statement, which reflects his belief in Western superiority and its leadership, as well as his faith in science to provide the tools to shepherd the global South into adopting modern family planning practices, effectively reinforced the co-constitutive relationship between science and Western imperialism.

Physicians who took on the task of developing IUDs readily identified with this biopolitical and geopolitical mission that Rockefeller promoted in support of their scientific activities. Lazar Margulies, inventor of the Gynekoil IUD and the recipient of the first IUD research grant from the Population Council, told colleagues that a 1958 lecture about "the dire consequences of overpopulation and the urgent necessity for large-scale conception control" had motivated him "to search for a simple, inexpensive, and reliable, permanent contraceptive that could be applied and removed easily."[34] In the journal *Obstetrics and Gynecology,* Charles H. Birnberg and Michael Burnhill, the inventors of the Birnberg bow IUD, asserted that gynecologists must exert their influence by supporting programs of research and development in areas that would further the cause of reducing the relentless pressure of rapidly growing populations. In the same article, they reviewed the status of the IUD and presented it as the most favorable method available for family planning programs.[35]

In an interview with historian James Reed, statistician Christopher Tietze, known for his work on the large-scale multinational clinical trials of the IUD, recalls the enthusiasm that surrounded the contraceptive device in its early days of development at the Population Council: "This was something you could do to the people rather than something people could do for themselves. So it made it very attractive to the doers."[36] As scientists and physicians, IUD advocates knew that the device was not yet perfect. They nonetheless pursued the idea that the global population problem had a technological solution. They reasoned that since men and women of the global South were incapable of regulating their own fertility, a technology that takes control over their bodies for them would best address the ostensible need to regulate population growth in the global South. IUD developers felt free to test their innovations in women in the name of human welfare. Searching for the ideal technology, while producing authoritative knowledge regarding intrauterine contraception, these researchers in effect took on the role of producing technoscientific biopower.

The Biopolitical Script of a "Birth Control for a Nation"

A "birth control for a nation," which providers could use to "do to the people," was imaginable only when that population was constructed as lacking agency. As historian Andrea Tone points out, the masses were rendered passive vessels of this birth control device and exploitable in many ways for a larger cause.[37] And as Anni Dugdale illustrates, the "unmotivated" and "submissive" "third world women" were coproduced with the "population-control IUD."[38] IUD supporters also actively characterized the masses as different from individuals in an attempt to differentiate their product from the pill. Alan Guttmacher's letter to the chairman of G. D. Searle, the first pharmaceutical company to market the oral contraceptive, epitomizes how population control advocates characterized the relationships of users to the technology to garner support for the IUD: "The big difference is that the IUD's are not as effective as the pill in preventing conception. If Mrs. Astorbilt, or Mrs. Searle or Mrs. Guttmacher gets pregnant while wearing an IUD, there is quite a stink. . . . However, if you reduce the birth rate of an unprotected segment of the Korean, Pakistanian, or Indian population . . . this becomes an accomplishment to celebrate."[39]

In contrast to Western white middle-class wives who were presumed to be capable of and entitled to take responsibility for managing their own fertility, IUD users of the global South were represented in terms of aggregate birthrates and as racialized, regionalized, and disindividualized populations. By segregating this population from Western consumers, IUD supporters carved out the need for an imposable technology.

Disindividualizing these users had harmful implications. First, accidental pregnancies in non-Western individuals were not considered critical as long as the contraceptive method suppressed overall birthrates. Moreover, and perhaps more gravely, the infections and consequential infertility that IUD insertions occasionally caused were often trivialized. Although not all physicians believed it wise to indiscriminately insert the device in all women and some recommended systematically excluding patients with certain preconditions, these considerations were significantly downplayed during the first international conference on the IUD in 1962.

The transcript of this conference indicates that during a discussion, one of the participants suggested that women might believe the IUD caused existing infections that later turned serious, and therefore it might be prudent to screen out at-risk patients in order to avoid any blame being placed on the device. Guttmacher opposed the idea. He pointed out that elaborate knowledge of the patient's previous and current health conditions as prerequisite would not only make IUD insertion a more time-consuming job, but it would be unrealistic because "in villages of India one would have a hard time getting a meaningful history as to whether or not [a woman has had] an infection."[40] Worrying about potential risks to individual women was contradictory to the larger objective for Guttmacher, who declared: "We dare not lose sight of our goal—to apply this method to large populations."[41] Agreeing, Robert Willson, the chair of obstetrics and gynecology at Temple University, went so far as to say: "How serious is [an intrauterine infection that ends up with a hysterectomy and surgical removal of both ovaries]? Not very. Perhaps we have to stop thinking in terms of individual patients and change our direction a bit."[42]

These discussions served to solidify the priority that developers placed on indiscriminate mass insertion as the mode of governance over women's bodies. In the same letter to G. D. Searle & Company, Guttmacher wrote: "No contraceptive could be cheaper, and also, once the damn thing is in, the patient cannot change her mind." Prejudices against women of the global South stripped them of the rights, trust, and reproductive control granted to Western white middle-class women. In the interest of reducing the aggregate fertility rate, individual health was rendered dispensable for racialized, classed, regionalized, and essentially dehumanized IUD users.

Conceptualizing women in the disindividualized aggregate allowed developers to reduce them to the function of their reproductive organ as the most prominent element involved on the assembly line of fertility control. IUD researchers turned their attention to fine-tuning what "the damn thing" did inside the uterus. Consequently studies of biopolitical subjects of the "birth control for a nation" concentrated on female physiology—more specifically, how uteruses responded to the device.

The Colonization of Women's Bodies and the Search for the Perfect Device

Whereas oral contraceptive developers had some theoretical knowledge of how a pill prevented pregnancy, how an IUD worked was a "mystery" to its researchers working with the Population Council in the 1960s.[43] Although there was an abundance of medical studies on uterine pathologies, studies of a normal uterus relevant to IUD use were scarce. In this setting of vast uncertainty, the uterus became akin to an unknown territory waiting to be explored with an IUD. Just as colonial science generated knowledge concerning colonial subjects that would be used to rule over them, IUD researchers investigated the "IUD-holding uterus" as a way to extend their influence to the "underdeveloped" regions of the world.

Researchers were keen to develop an IUD that would most effectively prevent pregnancy. In search of an ideal body-technology relationship, they invented various models of IUDs of different shapes and sizes, used X-rays to visualize how devices fit and filled the uterus, took measurements of uterine cavities, and competed against each other to create an overall superior device. Biologization of users and standardization of the uteruses that accompanied these research activities facilitated the removal of agency from individual IUD users. Close analyses of the scientific discourse and practices uncover how this was accomplished in the context of neocolonialism.

Tinkering with Design

Early IUDs were made of metal rings with a few exceptions such as the plastic Ota ring. The availability of flexible plastic enabled IUD researchers and producers in the 1960s to make and experiment with devices of various sizes, shapes, and surface areas. By altering the size, shape, and material of the device, they attempted to find a model that occupied the uterine cavity in some ideal way that would simultaneously reduce the pregnancy rate, expulsion rate, bleeding, and pain. By the 1970s, at least forty different experimental models made from a wide range of materials including plastic, silver, stainless steel, and silkworm gut were available (figure 2.1).[44]

Researchers hypothesized that it was important to find a version that would fit uteruses of various sizes and shapes well. They generally accepted the idea that a device that was too large in comparison to the uterus would cause more discomfort and get pushed out by uterine contraction more

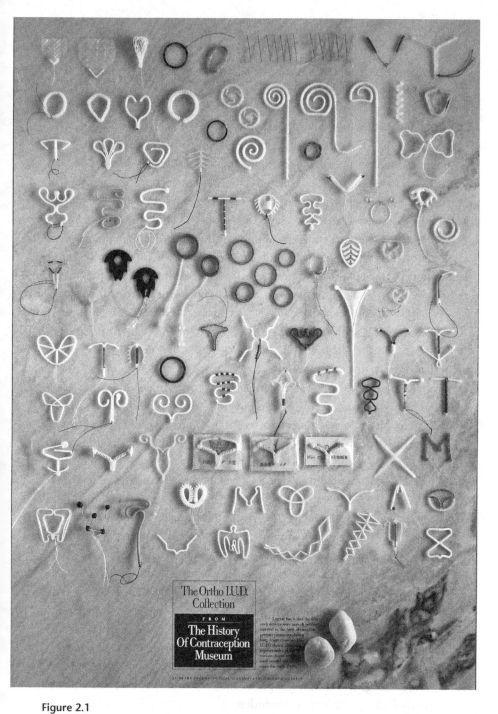

Figure 2.1

This poster shows the variety of IUDs developed since the 1920s in search of a design that best "fits" the uterus. Reprinted with permission from the Dittrick Medical History Center, Case Western Reserve University.

often, and that a device that was too small was more likely to permit pregnancy or migrate downward in the uterus and slip out.[45] Inventors often tested many different sizes of their particular design in order to determine which yielded the best overall outcome.

"Filling up" the uterus was also speculated to be important. The once popular double-S-shaped Lippes loop, invented by Jack Lippes in 1960, was designed based on the idea that a device that corresponds to the shape of the triangular organ would maximize its effectiveness by filling the uterine cavity "in a stable manner."[46] Hugh Davis, who invented the Dalkon Shield several years later, expressed similar ideas that the reason pregnancy rates were lower with larger spirals and loops was that these devices resulted in "better coverage of the endometrial surface" and that the higher pregnancy rate of the round stainless steel ring device was due to the "inadequate coverage of the endometrial cavity."[47] As I elaborate later, Davis created his device so that it achieved a large area of contact with the uterine surface.

Visualizing Uterine Occupation

Visually examining how well the IUD covered or occupied the uterine cavity to protect the uterus from pregnancy was one way in which researchers tried to quantify the relationship between body and technology. In order to investigate the correlation between the device's location in the uterus and the occurrence of pregnancy, expulsions, and side effects, Michael Burnhill and Charles Birnberg took seventy X-rays of uteruses containing six different sizes of the Birnberg bow. They calculated what they called the "ratio of occupancy" that the IUD achieved and found that in half of the patients X-rayed, "the device occupied more than 75 percent of the fundus."[48] They warned that "a silent downward migration of the device may leave large areas of the endometrial cavity *unprotected* by the contraceptive device," and hence "the mere presence of an [IUD] within the endometrial cavity gives no assurance of adequate fundal coverage to afford a good contraceptive effect."[49] IUD developers were unable to detect the behavior of the devices once they were inserted in the uterus. Hence visual observation using X-rays and calculating the occupied uterine area provided some concrete knowledge about how the device behaved and enabled researchers to hypothesize how the uterus responded.

The most elaborate work along these lines was done by Ibrahim Kamal, who spent fourteen years taking more than one hundred X-ray pictures, which he published in his 1979 book, *Atlas of Hysterographic Studies of the "IUD-Holding Uterus."*[50] The book is filled with X-ray images of the glowing shapes of IUDs superimposed on triangular white shadows of uteruses staged against a dark background (figures 2.2, 2.3, and 2.4). Kamal provides narratives of these images, noting that one of the uteruses became "very irritable" because it was too small compared to the device, which led to spotting and a "severe colic."[51] Another uterus was so large that the device became "loose and lost," or "disoriented and displaced," causing painless bleeding and resulting in a "cavity occupation [that is] incomplete."[52] He points out that when the device was observed to "fit snugly against the various borders of the uterine cavity," covering it completely and forming a "harmonious fit relationship," it was less likely to cause bleeding and pain or be expelled.[53] He characterized this result as the "ideal uterus-device relationship" in which the IUD-holding uterus was "symptomless."[54] Fellow IUD investigators praised the systematic medical gaze Kamal cast on women's bodies as one that advanced their research and would contribute to the device's effectiveness.[55]

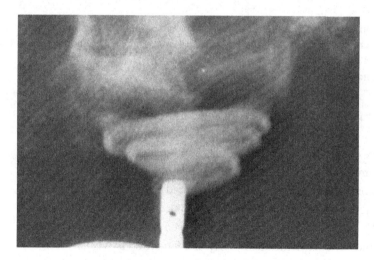

Figure 2.2
An X-ray figure of an IUD-holding uterus. Ibrahim Kamal labeled this image the "irritable uterus." He writes: "This is a small-sized uterus containing a Lippes loop C. . . . Severe colic necessitated early closure [first week] of the case" Kamal (1979, 25). Reprinted with the permission of IDRC, http://publicwebsite.idrc.ca.

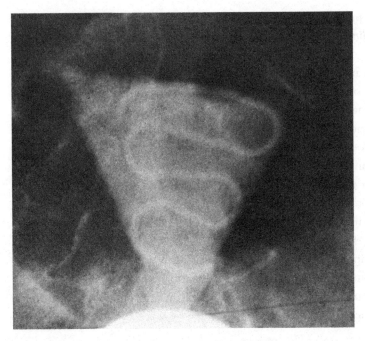

Figure 2.3
Kamal's caption reads: "A large triangular cavity containing a Lippes loop C. The loop lies 'loose and lost' in the cavity. Fundal coverage and cavity occupation are incomplete" Kamal (1979, 26). Reprinted with the permission of IDRC, http://publicwebsite.idrc.ca.

Visualization has been a powerful apparatus of colonization over women's bodies. When the first vaginal speculum, invented in 1845, "[threw] an abundance of light into the vagina and around the womb," the tool became an "instrument that would help organize the uncharted female landscape." Its inventor Marion Sims, who experimented with his device on slave women, pictured himself as an "explorer . . . [viewing] a new and important territory."[56] In a similar manner, X-rays allowed IUD developers to expose, explore, and conquer the hidden cavity of a female body. Visually and discursively representing the spatial area that one attempts to occupy and regulate is also reminiscent of the use of cartography by imperial powers in the eighteenth and nineteenth century. For example, maps rendered visible the lands Europeans had secured and, by drawing borders and accumulating knowledge about the place, they made territorial occupation and European governance over foreign land an actuality.[57] Kamal's and Birnberg's X-ray

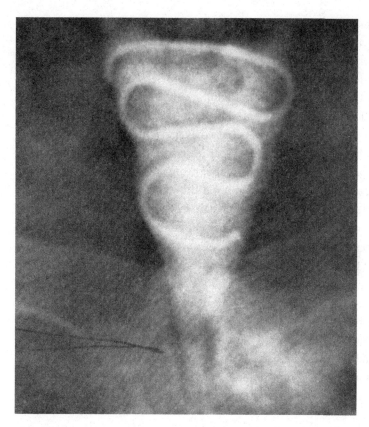

Figure 2.4
Kamal describes this image as a "harmonious fit relationship." The caption reads: "The loop is well oriented in the frontal plane; the fundus is totally covered with the base of the loop; the cavity is totally occupied; the edges of the loop fit snugly against the lateral walls" Kamal (1979, 15). Reprinted with the permission of IDRC, http://publicwebsite.idrc.ca.

pictures and narratives similarly revealed the concealed secrets of the relationship between the uterus and the IUD, and by visualizing the occupancy
of the organ by the device, they enabled the device's reign over the uterus.
According to Jane Carruthers, colonizers' maps served as a "visible way of
securing settler domination and providing conceptual reality in advancing
the formation of . . . a modern nation-state." X-ray visualization similarly
offered a way to identify the spatial coverage achieved by the IUD and
conceptualize technological rule over the uterus. A 1974 Lippes loop advertisement epitomizes this relationship by presenting a drawing of the device
occupying a uterus, "proving ground," as the ad's caption reads (figure 2.5).

The mission that the neo-Malthusian scientists who investigated the
"IUD-holding uterus" took was not so different from that of early colonizers who explored exotic places: both were attempting to extend governance over foreign lands in order to ensure global economic expansion and
stability. By producing knowledge about colonial land and subjects, colonial scientists helped increase European influence over foreign territory.
By visualizing and describing the IUD's effect over the otherwise hidden
uterus, X-ray imagery created "knowledge" of women's bodies, allowing
IUD researchers to envision control over the "native" woman's womb and,
by extension, over the "native land," upon which economic development
and modernity were to be built and maintained.

"Angry Uterus," Fears, and Desires

Although it was an ideal contraceptive method in theory, IUDs caused a
considerable number of problems in practice, including accidental pregnancies with the device in situ, spontaneous expulsions, scores of requests
for removal due to pain and bleeding, and penetration of the uterine
wall.[58] When IUDs failed, their developers, perhaps due to bewilderment
or frustrations that their innovations were not working as they had envisioned, often explained that the uterus was rejecting the insertion of the
foreign body. Sometimes they described expulsions as the ring "escaping"
the uterus, often undetected by the patient and followed by unwanted
pregnancy. However, scientists more commonly attributed the expulsion
problem as the act of an "angry uterus" that was "sending a message" by
contracting itself and expelling the device.[59]

Sometimes researchers blamed the uterus for being too pathological to
conform to the terms of the insertion. One inventor, for instance, labeled

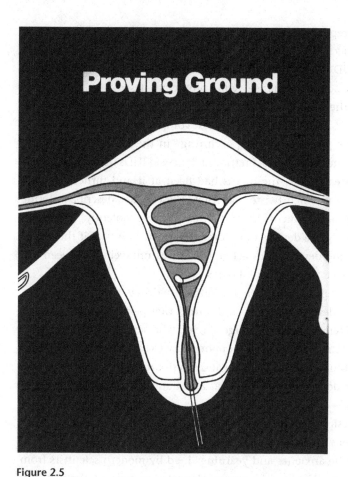

Figure 2.5
This advertisement of the Lippes loop by Ortho Pharmaceutical Corporation in New Jersey appeared in medical journals during the 1970s. It was accompanied by a headline that reads: "Any IUD that wants to prove its value has to prove it in the uterus." The visual representation shows how the device "fills" and occupies the uterus completely. (Ortho Pharmaceutical Corporation, *Journal of Reproductive Medicine*, 1974).

uteruses that repeatedly expelled devices "habitual ejecters": the X-rays showed an "incompetent internal os (opening)" that was "incapable" of keeping the IUD in place. But organic responses of the uterus were often interpreted as active resistance. One physician described spontaneous expulsions as the uterus's "ejective response" to the presence of an intra-uterine object.[60] Another described users' complaints of side effects as a sign of "uterine protest" that was occurring "in the form of cramps and bleeding." Yet another, who had retrieved damaged IUDs from her patients, explained: "In each case, the uterus had been at it and turned the ring into a figure eight which twisted on itself." Researchers described uterine contractions and movements as the uterus "reacting violently" and being "restless," causing the devices to become deformed. It was as if the uterus was attacking the device or an active battle was unraveling between the developers' devices and women's bodies. [61]

Ann Fausto-Sterling argues that scientists' writings provide a window into the "fears, desires, longings, and terrors that perfuse [their] works"[62] For example, French scientist George Cuvier, who scrutinized the physiology of Sarah Bartmann, took every opportunity to categorize the South African native woman as different from and inferior to white women, thereby dispelling any doubts about the racial and national superiority of white Europeans.

Both the desire to maintain the legitimacy of colonial rule and fear of losing the ruler's status are reflected in Cuvier's scientific work. Similarly, we can glean the anxieties and yearnings held by modern scientists from their work on the IUD-holding uterus. Their design concept aimed at fill-ing up the uterine cavity and forbidding expulsion mirrors their desire to colonize native women's bodies and "protect" the world from their preg-nancies. The X-ray cartography of IUD occupation parallels colonizers' use of maps to make real their dominion over a foreign territory: it shows how some scientists attempted to visualize and narrate the device's command over the physical space of the organ. Simultaneously, scientists articulated their uneasiness toward device failures. Their interpretation of users' physi-ological reactions to their devices suggests that they sensed an antagonistic relationship between themselves and the women who "reject," "eject," and "protest" the insertion of foreign objects and "resist" their neo-Malthusian agenda. Uterine resistance thus corresponded to native revolts against colo-nization. Researchers' rhetoric is also permeated with notions that women's bodies are close to "nature"—instinctual, irrational, and therefore difficult to control. Fear of fertile native bodies getting out of control and the desire to rule over them are implicit in these modern contraceptive researchers' scientific activities and theorizing.

Creating the Standardized Uterus

Physicians who probed IUD users' bodies often sidestepped consideration of individual women, viewing them instead as "the population." By personifying uterine responses, the scientific discourse effectively relocated individual women's agency to the reproductive organ and thus further contributed to the disindividualization of IUD users. Standardizing the anatomy of the already disindividualized mass of women users was another technique devised to construct a workable relationship between the uterus and the device.

Human uteruses are generally cone shaped, but they vary in size considerably and in terms of how wide, narrow, long, or short the triangular forms are. In fact, much of the inventing of IUDs depended on guesswork because no systematic studies of normal uterine cavity dimensions had been conducted before 1964. Hugh Davis, the inventor of the Dalkon Shield, and his collaborator, Robert Israel, addressed this problem by taking measurements of twenty silicone rubber casts of "fresh uterine specimens, removed by vaginal hysterectomy."[63] They plotted the measurements on a graph according to the widths of the top and the middle of the triangular uterus. The graph visually communicated the notable variation in "normal" uterine sizes—the largest uterus (37 millimeters) was more than twice as wide as the smallest one (15 millimeters). It also showed that the leading IUD models, the Margulies spiral and the Lippes loop, were larger than most of the twenty-five uteruses, while the stainless steel ring was about the same size as the cluster of smaller uteruses.[64]

Confirmation of variations in the size of the female reproductive organ posed a dilemma for the scientists, who believed that the IUD must "fit" or "fill" the uterus. Howard Taylor, who chaired the 1964 second international conference on the IUD, pointed out: "Dr. Davis's paper . . . raises the interesting question of whether there is an optimum ratio between a device's size and the variable uterine area." "This would raise great difficulties," he continued, "if a patient had to be fitted individually."[65] A few decades earlier, Margaret Sanger had given up on the diaphragm for the same reason: a method that requires a trained practitioner to screen women for health problems and fit them with devices appropriate for their particular cervical anatomy was impractical for broad distribution. The diaphragm was abandoned for an additional reason: Sanger believed that a contraceptive method that relied on individual users' initiative was counterproductive for her goal to restrict the birthrates of the underprivileged. The IUD eliminated the need for user involvement. But Taylor and others questioned the practicality of caring for each patient when their ultimate goal was to insert IUDs en masse and achieve fertility limitation on a large scale.

Instead of pursuing the idea of fitting each individual uterus with an appropriately sized device, Davis and Israel opted to create a device that "correspond[s] to the midrange of fundal dimensions."[66] With the idea of an "accommodative design" in mind, Davis started evaluating a shield design device in the Department of Gynecology and Obstetrics at the Johns Hopkins Hospital.[67] In his 1971 book, Davis shows the Dalkon Shield on a similar graph plotted with measurements taken from fifty uteruses (figure 2.6). The shield is shown on the graph as corresponding with the greatest number of uterine samples while the Lippes loop and the Saf-T-Coil are shown lying outside the average range.[68] Using a visual narrative, Davis conveyed the sense that the shield was somehow better suited for an average uterus than other models.

Davis's book also features photographs of commercially available IUDs laid on top of a triangle representing the "average uterine cavity size" of women who have had children (figure 2.7). The shield is shown to fit perfectly inside the borders of the triangle, and readers are told that "the flexibility and shape of the shield make it compatible with a broad range of uterine cavity size . . . making the overall performance of this second generation IUD distinctly superior."[69] Meanwhile, other common devices are shown as bigger or smaller than the triangle and described as being too "bulky" or too small, and thus unsatisfactory in one way or another.

The visual tactics Davis employed made the Dalkon Shield device appear "ideal" or somehow "accommodative" of the considerable variation in uterine size. Instead of fitting the IUD to the uterus, he co-configured his device with the "standard" uterus, which was created by averaging fifty distinctly shaped and sized uteruses.[70] These acts of extracting, measuring, and averaging the uterus rendered the recipient of the IUD a knowable entity. Standardizing the uterus erased anatomical variation among women and

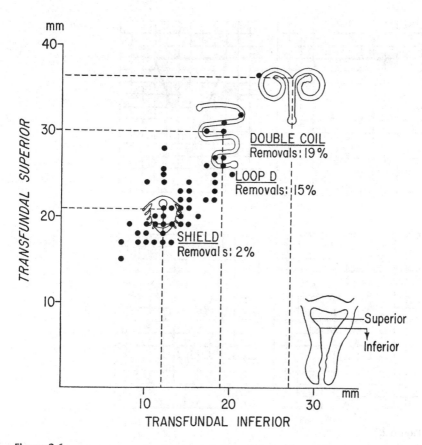

Figure 2.6
This graph represents the Dalkon Shield as corresponding to the majority of sample
uterine measurements, yielding a low removal rate (2 percent). It also shows other
models as being larger than most uterine measurements, resulting in high removal
rates of 15 to 19 percent. Davis (1971, 86). Reprinted with permission. Hugh Davis.
Intrauterine Devices for Contraception. (Williams and Wilkins, 1971).

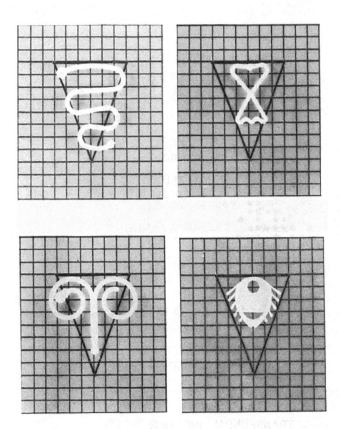

Figure 2.7
These are some of the figures that appeared in the appendix of Hugh Davis's book.
Juxtaposing various devices against a triangle that represents the "average" uterine
cavity size, Davis shows that most IUD models are "too bulky" or "too small" to
achieve optimal results. The Dalkon Shield is shown to fit the average uterus perfectly. Comments for the Dalkon Shield read: "The flexibility and shape of the shield
make it compatible with a broad range of uterine cavity size. Excellent retention
is accomplished in a unique way: because of its configuration, when the shield is
subjected to lateral compression, it buckles out of plane, utilizing the forces of uterine contraction to resist expulsion. The central membrane of this device enhances
endometrial surface contact, making pregnancy protection among young, highly
fertile women particularly good. . . . The shield combines low pregnancy rates, low
expulsion rates and low medical removal rates, making the over-all performance of
this second generation IUD distinctly superior" Davis (1971, 151). Reprinted with
permission. Hugh Davis. *Intrauterine Devices for Contraception.* (Williams and Wilkins,
1971), Appendix A, "Major Intrauterine Devices: Design, Performance Data, and
Availability."

universalized the bodies of the masses. Researchers' exclusive interest in the uterus had already displaced women's agency in favor of their biology. Homogenizing their bodies further muted their individuality and agencies. The standardized uterus thus advanced a technoscientific form of biopower by normalizing the relationship between the body and technology.

Overzealous Colonization and Violence against Women

Davis's and others' emphasis on an ideal configuration for the occupation of the uterus overshadowed any considerations about the health risks and physical discomfort their invasive devices imposed on women. An ultimate zealous endeavor to colonize the womb is represented by a device designed by Boston physician Herbert Horne. His invention was to be stapled onto the upper uterine wall in order to prevent expulsion and came with an inflatable balloon that would fill up the uterus. Citing Horne's patent, historian Andrea Tone disparages the IUD as "violence by design."[71] Although his device was never manufactured, other IUDs that focused on occupying the uterus and avoiding expulsion inflicted tangible violence on women.

The infamous Dalkon Shield was flat and wide because Hugh Davis hypothesized that low pregnancy rates would be achieved by increasing the total surface area of the plastic that would be in contact with the uterine wall.[72] But he seriously underestimated or underplayed the increased irritation and pain users experienced due to the additional contact. Davis also appended crab-like legs along the edges of his shield-shaped device to inhibit the device from migrating downward in the uterus and being expelled. This created a dangerous situation, where uterine contractions that would have ejected other devices made the shield embed itself in the uterine wall instead.[73] The M-device and the Majzlin spring were also designed with similar mechanisms to prevent expulsion. These metal devices, which sprang open inside the uterus so that they would become too wide to be pushed out through the cervix, were often extremely difficult to remove. The FDA eventually banned the Majzlin spring in May 1973, three years after the agency first received complaints about the device[74]

It has been well documented that the Dalkon Shield brought considerable misery to users in the United States—heavy bleeding during long periods, considerable cramping throughout the duration of use, and intense abdominal and lower back pain due to undetected cervical and uterine infections—rendering numerous women sterile and killing at least fifteen.[75] Russel Thomsen confirmed this from a physician's point of view in his testimony to the congressional hearing on IUD safety in 1973. He stated he had seen "women faint following . . . Dalkon Shield insertion," and many of his patients, who anticipated severe pain during the removal of shields and Majzlin springs, requested being "put to sleep."[76] Another doctor also described Dalkon Shield removal as "the most traumatic manipulation ever perpetrated upon womanhood."[77]

Violence against women was also metaphorically wielded through the discourse of war on population and hunger, which was juxtaposed against the cold war and later the war in Vietnam. Although the IUD had initially been considered to be the most promising "ammunition" for the war on population, by the time the United States was fighting in Vietnam, it was apparent that such an expectation was not met due to the large number of users abandoning the device. Matthew Connelly quotes an executive director of the Association for Voluntary Sterilization, who, while pushing for surgical sterilization, declared: "Although the IUD is another weapon in the war against hunger, its effective firepower in destroying the enemy is limited by its 40% failure rate. . . . It is hoped that we Americans will not lose the war on hunger by supplying the troops with blank cartridges, instead of calling for artillery strikes."[78] The enemy to be struck was the female fertile body. Immersed in combat metaphor, women were readily conceptualized as legitimate targets of violent assault. Describing the Population Council's approach, Colville Deverell, the director-general of the International Planned Parenthood Federation and a thirty-year veteran of Great Britain's Colonial Service, wrote, "The most effective procedure is usually to *attack* women in the post partum stage."[79] In addition to the imperialist neo-Malthusian logic that conceptualized women as disindividualized and exploitable masses, the war mentality served as a lubricant for coercive and semicoercive procedures administered on women of the global South.

The metaphor of war was also used in India, a country fighting its border nation Pakistan and where an aggressive IUD campaign took place. As India's minister of planning put it, population growth was "the enemy within the gate. . . . It is war that we have to wage." He continued with a remark intended to justify sacrifices: "As in all wars . . . some will get hurt."[80] India's Ministry of Health directed states to set targets and concentrate on densely populated areas. Women who agreed to accept IUDs or surgical sterilization were offered payment, and doctors were given incentives to perform these procedures. Some doctors reportedly inserted IUDs in half of postdelivery women.[81] "Loop squads" were dispatched to meet ambitious targets. Follow-up care was poor, and since complications were underreported, we do not know exactly how many women were victimized or suffered health problems as a result. No doubt a significant number of them became casualties of the Indian war on population in which the IUD was conceived to be a weapon. As feminist theorists have argued, metaphor is not just metaphor; it can have material consequences.[82]

Concentrating on the efficacy of the device and disregarding possible adverse health effects in favor of mass insertions amounted to additional violence against all women by faulty medical practices. As noted earlier, the consensus at the 1962 international conference on the IUD was that it was impractical to screen out patients with potential health risks if this contraceptive method was to be an effective tool for population control. Indiscriminate insertions would have introduced pathogens already present in the vagina to the normally sterile uterus, increasing the possibility of infections in the upper reproductive tract. Yet researchers failed to set careful criteria for insertions at the early stage of the introduction of this contraceptive method in both the global North and South. In addition, most insertion mechanisms originally involved pushing the plastic into the uterus from the inserter, which made it prone to perforating the uterine wall. American women did complain to their doctors about serious discomforts; however, many physicians were oblivious to the possibilities of infection and failed to diagnose it appropriately. Some were blatantly sexist: they dismissed the pain women were experiencing as a psychological reaction to a normal side effect and refused to remove the device.[83] Feminist authors have documented a number of testimonies in which women suffered permanent sterility due to IUD-related infections that went untreated for too long. Although personal accounts of women in the global South are rare, we can only imagine how much worse the situation must have been in regions where medical care was more difficult to access. By the mid-1960s, reports of adverse effects began coming in from overseas trial sites, but it was not until injuries sustained by American consumers became a public issue during the 1970s that IUD researchers began to address these dangers.

Quantification of IUD Users and the Universalization of the Female Body

While design tinkering efforts were underway, another major effort, the five-year clinical trial project known as the Cooperative Statistical Program (CSP), was conducted. This was an effort to evaluate the device's contraceptive efficacy. Developers anticipated that an extensive statistical study would not only prove the IUD to be an effective contraceptive method, but also give it scientific legitimacy and garner approval for the device from the medical community. Quantification also had the effect of making IUD users measurable, knowable, and therefore controllable biopolitical subjects. Meanwhile, converting women's experiences into statistical data obliterated critical social and personal differences that existed among users.[84] It furthered the production of a technoscientific biopower predicated on the existence of standardized machine-like bodies and knowledge about them.

The Cooperative Statistical Program
A significant agenda behind the CSP was to establish the IUD as a statistically proven modern scientific method, particularly since there was significant skepticism in the American medical community around intrauterine contraception. The Gräfenberg IUD had gained some popularity in Europe during the 1920s and 1930s.[85] Its German inventor, however, had to refrain from inserting his devices after migrating to the United States due to opposition from his colleagues. American physicians generally rejected the IUD because of its association with illegitimate sexual activities and for fear of infection and pelvic inflammatory disease.[86] A 1957 FDA survey showed widespread negative opinions among American obstetricians and gynecologists, leading to a conclusion that the distribution of IUDs should be condemned.[87] Under this circumstance, Alan Guttmacher predicted in his opening statement to the 1962 international IUD conference, "It is going to be extremely difficult to rehabilitate this method in the eyes of the medical profession throughout the world."[88]

Christopher Tietze, who later led the CSP, was convinced that before IUD supporters "can turn to the question of how this method can be used in mass distribution," they had to "[win] the support of . . . the medical profession."[89] To do this, they needed scientific data from a systematic study of the IUD. Tietze announced to his fellow conference participants: "Our first objective must be to convince our colleagues outside of this room that intrauterine contraception is a respectable medical procedure and not the devil's work. . . . Our planning for the next few years should be oriented toward careful clinical testing and not use on a large scale, even if this is our ultimate goal."[90] As chairman of the conference, Alan Guttmacher followed up by calling for a well-planned study on the device.

At this moment, some American physicians and Planned Parenthood officers who were attending the conference expressed ambivalence around the legal implications for experimenting with IUDs in the United States. They made subtle gestures toward conference participants from abroad, suggesting they might volunteer as test sites. After all, the first oral contraceptives had been tested a few years earlier in Puerto Rico and Haiti because developers found the countries to be legally favorable and because the islands were a "natural laboratory in the field": they provided ideal conditions that allowed experiments to be conducted without losing track of test subjects, whom researchers deemed as generally easy to convince to participate in medical trials.[91] It may have seemed commonsense for IUD trials to follow suit.

Population Council president Frank Notestein, however, stepped in to argue that the kind of criticism the pill developers received must be avoided:

Experimentation with intra-uterine contraceptives could be done in the countries where the legal situation is less complicated than in the United States. However, it is completely clear that a method, which is known but not used in the United States will meet very considerable resistance abroad. It will be alleged again that we, in the United States, experiment with other peoples. This was said about oral contraceptives. It was never true, but the story has very wide currency indeed and has been an obstacle. We have to face the legal situation of experimentation in the United States.[92]

Accordingly, Tietze was appointed to coordinate the multisite clinical trial program with the cooperation of mostly American investigators. The CSP extended from 1963 to 1968 and over that period evaluated five different IUDs: the Lippes loop, the Margulies spiral, the Birnberg bow, the stainless steel ring, and the Saf-T-Coil, added later. The final report included data on more than 31,000 women submitted by twenty-six clinical sites in the United States and three sites in other countries.[93]

As was common with previous attempts to study contraceptive effectiveness, many women stopped using the method or reporting to the clinics before the end of the trial, presenting major problems for the analysts. Researchers of the pill, who had also experienced high numbers of patient dropouts, reconciled the problem by converting women's duration of use into the number of menstrual cycles studied in total, which made the length of time each woman remained in the trial inconsequential.[94] Marcia Meldrum details the process by which Tietze found his way around the problem of the variance in the length of observation among IUD patients, many of whom were closed out of the study early. Tietze and his colleague Robert Potter devised the life table method to account for the relatively high discontinuation rates during the first few months of use. Under the assumption that women who disliked the method would drop out very early and the more "determined contraceptors" would remain in the trial longer, Potter developed a statistical formula that would "project the experience of a hypothetical couple using the method consistently over the entire period," while giving less weight in the computation for early quitters.[95] Although only 55 percent of the original subjects were still using the device at the end of the five-year study in 1968, the life table method allowed statisticians to adjust the results for the large number of early removals in calculating the pregnancy rates over the five-year period.

Using the life table method, the CSP yielded a pregnancy rate of 6.5 per 100 years for IUDs, which was low compared to diaphragms, spermicides, vaginal foams, and condoms and therefore acceptable by the standards at the time. When the FDA approved the pill for contraceptive use in 1960, it had been tested on only 1,600 women in the Caribbean field trial centers, covering 40,000 menstrual cycles.[96] Tietze's project included more than 31,000 women and 547,000 woman-months of use, allowing him to claim: "This project represents the first attempt in the history of fertility regulation to evaluate a new method from the time of its inception by the systematic analysis of pooled data, using uniform procedures and a sophisticated statistical approach."[97] As Meldrum concludes, "This statistically valid result established the medical legitimacy of the IUD and provided the justification for the Population Council's introduction of the device into fertility control programs around the world."[98] Successfully quantified and therefore scientized, the device became a legitimate medical device for the masses.

Collapsing Social Differences into Biological Sameness

Quantification of the IUD simultaneously had the effect of universalizing women as biologically similar beings. As Nelly Oudshoorn points out, substituting women in the pill trial with quantifiable menstrual cycles effectively erased differences among women.[99] She notes that researchers were quite aware that women were not uniform in terms of their resources and motivations and felt that testing with Caribbean women would allow them to demonstrate that uneducated women could use the pill as efficiently as educated women. Meanwhile, researchers also assumed that there were no fundamental bodily differences among women, which made it perfectly reasonable to test the drug in Caribbean women. When converted into number of menstrual cycles, Caribbean women became representative of all women, effacing social variations.

The CSP used mostly American clinic patients with the same assumption about women's physiological similarities and their social differences.[100] The IUD developers' intention was ultimately to target the masses in the global South, whom they clearly viewed as different from individuals or Western women. Yet they chose women in the United States for the tryout and generalized the test results to all women. As Oudshoorn aptly argues, representing pill users in terms of menstrual cycles implied "an abstraction from the bodies of individual women to the universal categories of physical process."[101] Transferring IUD users into women-months of use furthered the disindividualization of the population and device supporters' vision of mass fertility control.

Universalizing women as physically synonymous also concealed the process by which information about IUD use applicable to all females was created using data from particular kinds of women. Tietze and Potter's life table method depended on "determined contraceptors"—hypothetical users who through motivation, experience, and consistent use were able to achieve a statistically verifiable pregnancy rate. The contraceptive practices of couples who did not fit into the statistical model remained outside the analysis. As Anni Dugdale points out, through this procedure of creating statistical data, "the stories each woman has to tell of pain or pleasure, freedom from worry or increased worry as health deteriorates, are erased when the clinic participating in the trials fills in the follow-up form, reducing each woman's experience to a continuing trial participant or a closed-out case in one of the categories."[102] Reasons for discontinuations were recorded as medical, personal, or pregnancy. But detailed information was not systematically collected for the researchers to gain a good understanding of what led women to leave or be closed out of the trial. Individual experiences of bleeding, pain, and removal were immaterial to the goal of the researchers at this time. As Andrea Tone noted, "Viewing IUDs as birth control for the generic masses made it easier for gynecologists designing and inserting IUDs to deem irrelevant the unique attributes and varied responses of individual wearers."[103]

Assumptions about the universality of women's bodies allowed researchers to switch seamlessly from a certain type of ideal user to all women in their representations of IUD users. Although scientists originally targeted the masses, differentiating them from individuals, social differences among women were collapsed into a universal female body. Under the premise that all women's bodies are similar, the device was quickly disseminated to individuals, colonizing women's bodies in the global North. I explore the effects of such transformation in later chapters.

Shifting Terrain in the Late 1960s

In spite of the strong sense of purpose that guided the launching of IUD development projects in the early 1960s, the ground soon started to move beneath the developers, compelling them to make adjustments to their expectations, discourse, and research trajectories. Despite the development of an array of new IUDs in different sizes, shapes, surface areas, and other physical characteristics, high rates of user discontinuation of the method persisted. Studies comparing devices showed that design changes made only minor improvements; in fact, the performance differences among various clinical centers proved to be much more significant than among the models. "In spite of extensive clinical study of many IUD configurations and a reasonably good evaluation methodology," declared one of the researchers, "the effort to improve intrauterine contraception has proved 'expensive and frustrating.'"[104] After nearly a decade of inventing, devising, measuring, gazing, and experimenting, developers had to come to terms with the idea that some women simply could not tolerate IUDs. Physicians conceded that they could do very little but suggest to patients that they persist through the first few months until the uterus, they hoped, began to "accommodate the device and react less violently to its presence."[105]

Distribution efforts in developing nations also faced difficulties. The Population Council's Technical Assistance Division actively supported governments of the global South in implementing family planning programs by providing technical and financial assistance, donating large quantities of IUDs, and facilitating local manufacturing of the device. The council also obtained rights to provide royalty-free licenses for the manufacture and distribution of the Lippes loop in developing countries so that they could be procured locally and cheaply. As early as 1966, however, the developers began to see that the results were ambiguous. Council President Frank Notestein reported: "It is both curious and important to note that the year in which the first claims of successful reduction in birth rates could be made, thanks to the effectiveness of the IUD, was also the year in which some disillusionment with the IUD began to emerge."[106] On the one hand, he believed that the availability of the IUD convinced leaders in developing nations that "they had a method of sufficient promise to warrant the establishment of a major family planning service."[107] On the other hand, he admitted that the effort to distribute the IUD in developing nations had focused too much on the "ideal exercise" and paid "too little attention . . . to actual practices."[108]

The ideal exercise assumed that once a perfect device was invented, this one-time intervention method would achieve population control relatively easily. Under this presumption, scientific work had emphasized the physiological features of the device, while taking scant consideration of how social conditions and women's responses might affect use patterns in actual practice. As developers came to find, women who had been categorically conceived as passive recipients of the device exercised limited, but nevertheless important, agency. The council reported that users who were not informed of the heavy bleeding and pain that might accompany IUD use insisted on removal when they experienced these effects, and the council lamented that "dissatisfied women have spread adverse gossip and encourage[d] others to discontinue."[109] While it dismissed women's production of user-based knowledge as "gossip," the Population Council was nevertheless compelled by the negative impact of information spread by women to rethink its approach and acknowledge that more attention needed to be paid to women's satisfaction.

In short, the early dissemination efforts of the IUD yielded mixed results. This can be observed, for example, in the contrast between disappointments in India and perceived successes in Korea and Taiwan. As the first government in the global South to institute an official population policy in 1952, India received significant attention and funding from the Western population establishment, at the same time that it also became a source of tremendous frustration for neo-Malthusians. The Indian government's effort to widely enforce fertility control was hampered by state health departments that did not share their goals and the shortage of doctors and hospitals for sterilization operations. The Indian Health Ministry was slow to come on board with the adoption of the IUD, which compelled Sheldon Segal of the Population Council to smuggle IUDs into India by disguising them as Christmas ornaments to start a clinical trial there in 1964. After the Ford Foundation promised medical research as an incentive for conducting the test, a massive Lippes loop campaign was launched in the country. The council provided more than 1 million IUDs until a local factory was constructed.[110] Women were recruited and devices were inserted without much information given to the recipients. In order to meet ambitious targets, various questionable practices were put in place, including the "loop squads" and monetary incentives for doctors and IUD accepters.[111]

Although the recruitment was initially successful, programs began to falter as many women developed adverse effects. By 1972, only a negligible percentage of Indian women were using IUDs, and India as a whole had almost discontinued the program. Kumudini Dandekar explains that the unexpected bleeding raised "panic" among women who were not adequately informed.[112] When problems of bleeding and pain took their toll, some rural women made "their own decisions to get over their troubles" and removed the device themselves instead of going back to the clinic for help.[113] To the dismay of the Population Council, Indian women also convinced their relatives and acquaintances to remove their IUDs and not accept any new ones. Comparing the Indian IUD programs to those in East Asia, Dandekar and colleagues explain that India lacked the follow-up capacities for individual attention that should have been part of an IUD program. And since IUDs required good aftercare, they concluded, they could not be an appropriate method for the masses.

In contrast, South Korea and Taiwan became the poster children of the Population Council. Both countries received significant support from the council for their IUD programs while concurrently their birthrates declined.[114] The reasons for such regional differences are complex, and I address them only briefly here. Anni Dugdale points out that the medical authority in Taiwan was committed to the program and was prepared to allay women's fears induced by excessive pain and bleeding, whereas in India, the support of the local medical profession was not sufficiently garnered.[115] In general, factors such as being more secular societies, rising prosperity, literacy, and sharply visible limits of expansion due to the small geographical size of these states are believed to have worked in the favor of the East Asian countries.[116] The success of family planning programs also depends on an adequate institutional and clinical infrastructure and factors including political acceptability, government investment, availability of good-quality clinical services, women's status, and local culture.[117] South Korea, for example, had strong institutional support from the Planned Parenthood Federation of Korea founded in 1961.[118] The South Korean government was also one of the first in the world to adopt an official family planning program in 1962, launching the "Stop at 2" campaign.[119]

Although the East Asian countries were positive examples for the rest of the world from a neo-Malthusian perspective, their purported success inevitably involved problematic practices. To begin, post–World War II American neoimperialism in the region was built on prior Japanese colonialism that used Taiwan and Korea during the 1930s as testing grounds for an early version of a Japanese IUD. Although the extent of this device's distribution during colonial times is not known, it was in use again in Korea in the postwar period.[120] The South Korean government that followed a military coup in May 1961 was so strongly behind population growth reduction that it made Frank Notestein of the Population Council nervous about blatant abuse of state power over fertility control.[121] John DiMoia details how South Korean authorities enthusiastically embraced biomedicine as a means to control their own people. The Lippes loop campaign started in 1964 and lasted until 1968 with strong support from the Population Council. It spread loop users widely from urban to rural areas with mobile clinics that traveled to villages to provide one-time insertions. Over these four years, the loop was the primary vehicle of the Korean family planning program and was heavily promoted as a modern alternative to the social and economic problems of large families. Although the extent of abuse is contested, there was certainly potential for coercion. Due to the lack of follow-up care, many women were left with debilitating physical problems. Owing to the logistical difficulties in delivering IUDs to remote areas and the complications women experienced, which resulted in a large number of dropouts, the South Korean family planning program switched to using the pill more predominantly after 1968.[122]

Despite these ambiguous results, Population Council president Bernard Berelson held on to the hope for a technological panacea. In 1969, he said he still favored "research on a mass involuntary method with individual reversibility."[123] Echoing his sentiment and frustrated by India's slow progress, a Ford Foundation official proposed an imaginary contraceptive mist that could be sprayed from a plane flying over India, which could only then be neutralized by an annual antidotal pill prescribed to those who were deemed to be eligible for having children. Berelson wanted to take a host of measures to limit births, including "indoctrination via satellite television broadcast, the reversal of tax and housing benefits for families, and adding sterilizing agents to water supplies."[124] By the late 1960s, however, others, such as one senior World Bank official quoted by Connelly, had become uneasy about openly promoting "population control" because the term carried an "image of rich white north controlling the growth of the poor dark south" and because "those who are opposed to or suspicious of family planning [we]re all too ready to exploit [the negative impression]."[125] Indeed, by this time, skeptics from transnational and diasporic communities, such as African Americans in the United States, were starting to voice concerns over the imperialist and eugenicist nature of neo-Malthusian projects.

By May 1972, top leaders of the population establishment had recognized that mass IUD insertion programs had provoked resistance in South and East Asia, Tunisia, Haiti, and elsewhere. Ten years after hosting the first conference on the IUD, the Population Council was compelled to revisit the premise that population growth must be quickly curbed in order to avert global catastrophe, as well as to revise the conviction that there is a technological solution to excess fertility. In 1973, Berelson officially recognized that at least five competing approaches to dealing with population growth had emerged, including one that deemed population growth as a nonproblem because social and economic development would automatically induce fertility rate decline and one that criticized population reduction efforts as a neocolonialist project that sought to protect the interest of rich countries at the expense of poor ones.[126] Berelson explained that as interest in population control developed during the 1960s, "counterpositions" and "backlashes" had naturally developed against the notion that controlling population growth would solve or prevent a variety of social and political problems.[127] Various positions in favor of broad social and economic development, with demographic adjustment merely a corollary, emerged during this time, in part from poorer countries' suspicions of richer countries' motives behind supporting population limitation. Over the first decade of IUD revival, as international debates complicated the positions on population control, the monolithic "mission" that population control advocates envisioned became considerably muddled.

As the field of population studies transformed from a straightforward scientific issue to a larger political issue, the Population Council also had to revisit its technocentric approach. Initially it had conceptualized the population problem as something that would be easily addressed once developing countries' governments recognized it as such. The organization would then provide assistance in measuring demographic trends and delivering contraceptives. Armed with the IUD and programs prepared to train local demographers, the council imagined itself as an agent that provided a technical solution to a technical problem of population growth. As population studies transformed from a seemingly straightforward science to a field encompassing larger political issues, the council had to modify its approach.

The technocentric approach was also attenuated as the IUD proved not to be a panacea for the population crisis. The centrality of the IUD as the one-size-fits-all contraceptive solution to an obvious problem therefore was relatively short-lived in the minds of its advocates. The grants issued by the Population Council for IUD development, which had peaked at $500,000 in 1965, declined as quickly as it had increased.[128] Nevertheless, the IUD continued to hold an important position as a tested long-acting contraceptive, particularly since Norplant and Depo-Provera, the other long-term methods, also proved not to be ideal in all situations. The perceived importance of the IUD to family planning in the global South sustained the council's interest in the device and therefore its continued investment in it. For decades to follow, the organization was instrumental in developing the copper-bearing and hormone-releasing devices as well as improving the safety and acceptability of the contraceptive method and promoting its dissemination.

The IUD as Technoscientific Biopower

The paradigm of a technical solution to a technical problem turned out to be oversimplified for the global neo-Malthusian movement. Still, in the decades that followed, the IUD has played the role of the agent of biopower in a number of countries. China used it in the most draconian way in the state's one-child policy in the 1980s, requiring every woman to be inserted with a tamper-resistant stainless-steel IUD after giving birth to her first child.[129] Under an ambitious population policy instituted by General Suharto, Indonesia in the early 1980s reportedly rounded up women to be inserted with IUDs, sometimes at gunpoint if they resisted.[130] Postwar Vietnam is another place where the IUD has been used heavily in its national family planning program.[131]

The contraceptive method has also been mobilized in racially motivated fertility control programs in the United States. Elena Gutiérrez's study of sterilization abuse against Mexican and African American women at the University of Southern California's Los Angeles County Medical Center found that counselors aggressively recommended IUDs to minority mothers who had just given birth. What a medical student witnessed in the 1970s in this American hospital is remarkably similar to the factory-style insertions that impressed Alan Guttmacher earlier in Taiwan. Dr. Karen Benker remembers that the drive to insert IUDs was so great that instead of receiving a postpartum checkup, minority women "were merely placed on the table one after another and an IUD was popped into place."[132]

The lure of long-acting and permanent contraceptive methods remained strong for those who believed in making interventions to avert what they deemed as undesirable births. Reports from Mexico during the late 1990s suggest that indigenous women were targeted heavily to use the IUD and that medical staff were inserting IUDs without their knowledge or proper consent in women who had just given birth or had an abortion.[133] In the United States, CRACK (Children Requiring A Caring Kommunity), a nonprofit group that offers cash to drug addicts who agree to contraception, paid 671 women to be sterilized and 15 women to use long-term birth control by its fourth year in 22 cities nationwide between 1997 and 2000.[134] A 2002 news article reported that an eighteen-year-old mother, also a former methamphetamine user, received $200 from CRACK for being fitted with an IUD.[135]

These accounts confirm that this imposable device has been, and still can be, regarded as the technological solution to socially undesirable fertility. As Patrick Joyce put it, material things bear "conditions of possibility." Objects do not necessarily determine outcomes, but "they carr[y] a certain capacity for action, and built into them [are] certain kinds of agency."[136] For instance, diaphragms originally attracted birth control advocates in the 1930s because they enabled women to take control of their reproduction. They were perceived as a women-centered method that enabled users to exercise individual agency. This capacity of the diaphragm resurfaced when the pill's health risks began to surface in the late 1960s, only this time population control advocates rearticulated the barrier method as a safer contraceptive for middle-class and better-educated women who were capable of acting responsibly. In their new discourse, the pill was recommended to only those who "couldn't" or "wouldn't" use the diaphragm.[137] This example shows that the diaphragm once again embodied women-initiated reproductive control. Similarly, IUDs retain the capacity to exercise eugenicist and population control agendas. Although the ethics and discourses of fertility control have changed substantially since the 1960s and 1970s, these biopolitical scripts remain embodied by the device, thus preserving the possibilities for future practices of coercive and exploitative fertility control.

IUD developers from the 1960s had a clear political interest in regulating fertility to limit national and international population growth. In their hands, this contraceptive method emerged as a technology that was unambiguously biopolitical. This chapter demonstrated how this imposable device was co-constructed with users who were presumed to be unable or unwilling to contracept and a mode of governance that prioritizes mass insertions. Population control advocates' vision to make a large-scale technological intervention in the reproductive lives of the global South was buttressed by a prevailing discourse of overpopulation, neocolonialist mind-sets, and prejudices against underprivileged women of color. The discourse of the IUD constructed and effaced differences among women at the same time. It positioned the IUD as a contraceptive given to the masses, while user-controlled contraceptive methods were characterized as appropriate only for educated upper- and middle-class Western individuals. Constructing these hierarchies among women permitted them to strip prospective IUD users of individual agencies and view users as bodies en masse targeted for technological intervention. At the same time, scientific discourse removed agency from women by focusing exclusively on the performance of their reproductive organs. It also obscured social differences as it rendered all women as biologically similar for a one-size-fits-all contraceptive. Universalizing women depoliticized scientific work and made approaching women as a population easier. Issues of health risks and women's choice were largely muted in the early IUD discourse. Subsequent chapters illustrate how new concerns were accommodated by the discourse and the device was transformed into a politically versatile technology built on the foundation of technoscientific biopower elucidated in this chapter.

3 From the "Masses" to the "Moms": Governing Contraceptive Risks

I was looking forward to getting an IUD when I phoned the doctor at a local Planned Parenthood office in April 2002. So I was momentarily taken aback by the way she responded to my request for an IUD insertion. She immediately asked me whether I was married, and when I said no, she followed up with more questions: "Are you and your partner faithful to each other?" "How long have you been with this man?" "Are you and your partner committed to a long-term relationship?" and on and on. Why was she asking me such personal questions? I did not want her to refuse to give me my contraceptive method of choice. Fortunately, I recalled reading about screening out young promiscuous women because they were believed to be at a higher risk of contracting pelvic inflammatory disease (PID). Gathering my thoughts quickly, I volunteered some information: I was in my late thirties, had one child, and did not plan to have another one anytime soon. I added that even if I were to try to conceive in the future and experienced difficulties, I would not know if my advanced age or the IUD were to be blamed. With this assurance, the doctor agreed to insert an IUD in me.[1]

In retrospect, I was fortunate to find a willing doctor. In 2002, many physicians still believed IUD insertions were risky, and the number of prescriptions was low.[2] My exchange with this doctor exemplifies the kind of scrutiny over sexual relationships, age, number of children, and willingness to consent to risk that women still receive as a prerequisite to IUD insertions in the United States. IUD developers were initially reluctant to necessitate user screening, viewing it as counterproductive to their goal of population control. The contrast between the indiscriminate insertions of the 1960s and this current climate of careful identification of a user that the doctor deems appropriate is remarkable. Of course, forty years had passed by the time I was calling Planned Parenthood, and the geographical and social contexts were vastly different. Nevertheless, I note this contrast because it highlights how different women's bodies are managed differently for divergent reasons. The historical process that transformed the ideal users from the masses to the moms involved the reshaping and multiplication of biopolitical subjects, or kinds of bodies regulated by the IUD, in accordance with the transnational political economy.

This chapter charts how IUD researchers have engaged the issue of risk associated with contraceptive use since the 1960s. It illustrates how ideas about risk are co-constitutive with different implicated users, bodies, and modes of governance—or biopolitical scripts—that have emerged around this contraceptive method over the past five decades. As IUDs reached middle-class users in the mid-1960s, its developers were compelled to revise the concept of IUD users as a homogeneous mass because the U.S. social context introduced new concerns around contraceptive use that were not considered when IUD supporters were focusing on women in the global South. Departing from the view of users as uniformly underprivileged, undereducated, and excessively fertile women, or targets of population control, researchers on the device began to take into account differences in women in terms of their race, class, nationality, age, marital status, childbearing history, and sexual activity. IUD developers, who had once assumed that health risks associated with the device were negligible, also began to reconceptualize bodily and other risks in accordance with the shifting social and geographical contexts. Changing situations gave rise to concerns such as teen pregnancies, infections or other health complications, and lawsuits against medical practitioners and device manufacturers, while they produced different meanings of "risk" with various profiles of "risky" users. At the same time, certain "safe" bodies were differentiated from dangerous ones and presented as appropriate users of the device, which its researchers considered to be an inherently safe technology. Different modes of governance, or a range of strategies to discipline diverse female bodies to avoid risk, were formulated within the IUD discourse.

I begin with a story that is familiar to many readers in the United States: the Dalkon Shield fallout that began in the early 1970s and its aftermath that continued through the 1980s. The shield was created and distributed independent of the Population Council's efforts to establish the IUD as an acceptable contraceptive method. But the shield crisis became a pivotal point that drew the attention of IUD researchers to the issue of risk. I review the story of the shield first to contextualize the analyses of historical incidents and research activities that surrounded the public questioning of IUD safety. I then return to the 1960s to examine the initial introduction of the modern IUD to American women and why health risks were largely overlooked. Subsequently I turn to the Population Council's effort to develop the copper-bearing IUD, which overlapped with the rise of interest in teen pregnancy in the United States and later the downfall of the shield and the deteriorating reputation of IUDs in general. Then I investigate the post–Dalkon Shield crisis recovery stage, detailing the process by which IUD supporters rehabilitated the device through the reconstruction of a "safe" relationship between the body and technology. Finally, I provide an analysis of the relationships among multiple sets of implicated users that resulted from diversified development trajectories. I argue that the reproductive *choice* of women in the global North and the *control* over fertility in the global South became interlocked in the process of negotiating the acceptability of the IUD as a contraceptive method for women throughout the world.

The Dalkon Shield Tragedy and Its Aftermath

The American experience with IUDs cannot be told without a careful account of the Dalkon Shield. At least fifteen women died and thousands of others suffered life-threatening infections, miscarriages, sterilization before even having the chance to have children, and chronic pain as a result of wearing a device that was zealously marketed using false information.[3] I have chosen to keep my discussion of the shield relatively brief in this book—not to trivialize the matter but because several books have been dedicated to women's horrifying experiences with the device and the lawsuits. For detailed information on the shield, readers may turn to these writings.[4] Here, I summarize the key facts and briefly discuss the aftermath so that I can discuss retrospectively how the U.S. introduction of IUDs led up to the Dalkon Shield disaster, and to set the historical context for the discussions of how IUD development trajectories, including the reintroduction of the copper T IUD and the rewriting of IUD safety standards, were affected by the sheild's fallout.

A Story of Corporate Greed and Medical Neglect
The shield-shaped plastic device with spikes on the sides was invented in
1968 by Hugh Davis, director of the Family Planning Clinic at Johns Hopkins University, and his collaborators. A. H. Robins produced and sold the
Dalkon Shield between January 1971 and June 1974 in the United States.
Overseas distribution was halted in April 1975. Aggressive marketing,
sometimes employing misleading data, helped boost the shield's popularity. According to a third-party study, the actual pregnancy rate of the device
was five times as high as advertised. The company, however, consistently
dismissed unfavorable reports and complaints from physicians who had
seen a high frequency of pregnancies and complications among their patients and continued to promote the shield as a "modern," "superior," "second generation," and "safe" IUD.[5]

After the shield had been on the market for a couple of years, a few
physicians who had experienced serious complications among their patients went public with their conviction that the device posed a danger to
its users. Russel J. Thomsen, a medical doctor in Louisiana, was the first to
criticize the Dalkon Shield at a congressional hearing on May 30, 1973. Enticed by A. H. Robins's promotional campaign, he had inserted hundreds of
IUDs in patients, only to realize later that the devices inflicted tremendous
pain on many of them.[6] In the hearing, he used strong language in criticizing the contraceptive method. He condemned gynecologists who "carved
and twisted various metals, plastics and fibers into objects which they have
then inserted into the depth of trusting patients" and then subsequently
proclaimed to have invented "the perfect IUD."[7] He scolded the government for not regulating a medical device that had devastating effects on
women's health.

Word started to reach the general public when Morton Mintz wrote an
article for the *Washington Times* the next day titled, "Doctor Attacks IUD
Safety."[8] In December 1973 A. H. Robins finally reported four deaths related to the Dalkon Shield to the U.S. Food and Drug Administration (FDA).
Yet it took the company another six months before it mailed "Dear Doctor" letters, advising them to remove the shield from pregnant women. Six
months later, in June 1974, Donald Christian, whose patient got pregnant
with a Dalkon Shield in place and later died from an overwhelming infection, published a report in the *American Journal of Obstetrics and Gynecology*.
According to the information he collected, there had been five deaths of

pregnant IUD users and seven additional users who became severely ill with septic abortions; all but one from each category were Dalkon Shield users.[9] Both Thomsen and Christian called for a more rigorous evaluation and control of medical devices through FDA regulation. "Certainly," wrote Christian, "if there were five botulism deaths from one type of mushroom soup, the Food and Drug Administration would do more than put out a questionnaire."[10]

The FDA, however, did not act as promptly as one might expect, even after Planned Parenthood quickly recalled all Dalkon Shields following A. H. Robins's "Dear Doctor" letter. If the agency had swiftly ordered a recall of the shield, additional damage to women's health could have been prevented. During the hearing in August 1974, the agency recommended removing the shield from pregnant women but also said that shields being worn without complications need not be removed because "there is simply not enough evidence to convict or acquit the shield."[11] Although A. H. Robins had temporarily halted sales (and never resumed again) two months earlier in June, it had made no effort to warn women that the safety of the device was under investigation.[12] Not until a decade later, in October 1984, after numerous lawsuits, did A. H. Robins initiate a recall campaign that included a Dalkon Shield removal program for women who still wore them.[13]

According to the company's own estimate, 56 of every 100 IUDs inserted in the United States were the shield by the end of 1971, and by the end of 1973, the shield outnumbered the two leading rivals—the Lippes loop by two to one and the Saf-T-Coil by four to one. The company sold 4.5 million devices in eighty countries before halting sales. An estimated 2.2 million American women had the Dalkon Shield inserted. If we accept the 5 percent pregnancy rate, 110,000 American women would have gotten pregnant with the shield in place. The company's own conservative estimate in April 1985 was that 4 percent of Dalkon Shield wearers were injured, which amounts to 90,000 women in the United States. Soon after the controversy broke out, women started to sue A. H. Robins for their injuries, and a few won multimillion-dollar settlements. In 1985, a class action suit was filed against the company, and during the same month, A. H. Robins filed for bankruptcy to escape further financial damage.[14] The claimants, ultimately 300,000 of them, had to wait many years before receiving only limited compensation.[15]

The Aftermath

The Dalkon Shield fallout left a significantly dampened U.S. market for IUD distributors. In 1982, 7 percent of all contraceptive users used the IUD. That figure dropped to 3 percent in 1987 and 1 percent in 1992.[16] In numbers, IUD users decreased from 2 million in 1982 to 0.3 million in 1995.[17] In addition to the dwindling number of users, pharmaceutical companies experienced mounting costs of defending lawsuits, and obtaining product liability insurance became virtually unaffordable for them.[18] Because they were no longer profitable, major pharmaceutical companies discontinued their IUD products in the United States by 1986.[19]

The withdrawal of IUDs from the American market was a mixed blessing. If the FDA had recalled the Dalkon Shield sooner, thousands of women would not have faced major health problems. The disappearance of other models may have saved many underprivileged women from having the device imposed on them. Some users, however, had preferred the IUD to other forms of contraception.[20] As Adele Clarke points out, subtle forms of sterilization abuse can occur when access to other means of contraception is lacking.[21] Some of those who lost access to IUDs may have had to opt for (or, worse yet, may have been forced into) surgical sterilization.[22] Fear of lawsuits and the unavailability of liability insurance led doctors and clinics to refuse to insert IUDs even if they had the device in stock. Some doctors allegedly referred women to colleagues in Canada, where IUDs were still being sold, and Canadian family planning clinics reported inserting IUDs in women who came from the United States to request them.[23] Significantly, the withdrawal of the relatively safer models from the market in the mid-1980s was not out of concern for users but about protecting the profits of the companies and the providers from litigation. For women who preferred the method, the disappearance of IUDs from the market was equivalent to losing their contraceptive choice.

IUD Distribution in American Women in the 1960s

The Dalkon Shield case was particularly egregious. But it was also a predictable outcome of the historical trajectory of IUD development and its introduction to the United States at that historical moment. When the IUD was introduced to American women, developers were focused on overpopulation. Reflecting their focus on inserting the devices to prevent undesirable pregnancies in particular groups of women, the initial use patterns in the United States showed high rates of minority women users. The contraceptive method, however, was quickly adopted by those whom IUD developers considered "individual" patients, or middle-class white consumers whom they had originally ignored, believing that the pill was more adequate for this group. The assumption that this technology would be inserted indiscriminately on a large scale had led developers to underplay potential health risks. In effect, infections were inevitable under the insertion protocols that they had foreseen.

The CSP and the Domestic Masses

The Cooperative Statistical Program (CSP), the large-scale IUD clinical trial program initiated in 1963, involved mostly American collaborators, including a number of Planned Parenthood clinics and large inner-city hospitals, as well as private practice physicians. Hence, the first American women to be inserted with IUDs were subjects in this trial. While the goal of IUD development was to limit population growth in the global South, there was also an assumption that the device would be suitable for poor people everywhere. As Joanna Schoen notes, the national and global population programs had a number of parallels in the 1960s when family planning became an official U.S. government program to fight the "war on poverty."[24] Reflecting this trend, Alan Guttmacher in 1964 noted that IUDs had "tremendous and pertinent application" in "our own country among the least privileged elements, where motivation for family planning is limited."[25]

Poor Americans, who once had difficulty accessing contraceptives, quickly became targets of family planning. Health workers who served indigent clients readily started prescribing the pill, which was released a few years before IUDs were available.[26] Like the global population control advocates, however, some domestic officials believed that poor women were unwilling to prevent conception or unable to use the pill correctly. For example, a health director of North Carolina's Robeson County was quoted in a 1963 Raleigh newspaper saying, "I know these people and they don't take [the pills] like they ought to."[27] In his county, welfare officials decided to limit contraceptive offerings to the IUD in family planning programs aimed at "holding down the number of children born into poor families, especially those receiving welfare grants."[28] Similar to the zealous contraceptive distribution programs overseas, programs targeting indigent women in North Carolina neglected aftercare.[29]

During this time, population limitation practices implemented in former colonies were also transferred to the United States, continuing the neo-Malthusian movement on women in the diaspora. For instance, when population control enthusiast Dr. Antonio Silva moved from his public health post in Puerto Rico to Lincoln Hospital in the Bronx, New York, the sterilization rates of low-income Puerto Rican women in the neighborhood went up.[30] Within a social climate that approved restricting the reproduction of certain groups of women, IUD application in controlling the fertility of the domestic masses started almost immediately, in parallel with the global project of population control. Half of Planned Parenthood of America's 128 affiliates adopted the device by 1965, offering it to poor clients.[31] Not surprisingly, twice as many black women as white women used the IUD at this early stage.[32]

Commercial IUDs Reach Individuals

IUD developers initially paid little attention to "Western" women since they had characterized them as pill users in order to justify the need for a long-acting alternative method for national population limitation programs.[33] IUDs, however, quickly found their way to middle-class American women, facilitated by a breakthrough in the development of the oral contraceptive and its successful introduction to the U.S. market in 1960. Before the arrival of the pill, the physician's role in birth control was limited to fitting diaphragms. When oral contraception appeared as a prescription medication, physicians grasped the opportunity to take on the role of chief custodians of the new technology and heightened their professional authority as experts on the topic of fertility control.[34] Media attention to the pill removed social inhibitions of discussing birth control, and women who had been too shy to inquire about contraception started to request the pill from their doctors. By the time IUDs entered the market in the mid-1960s, the popularity of the pill had already prepared both doctors and patients to embrace this latest medical contraceptive.[35]

The financial success of the pill no doubt attracted entrepreneurs to this new contraceptive method as another possible business opportunity. By 1968, twenty-eight IUD models were known to the FDA, sixteen of them patented or with a distributor.[36] Among them, models such as the Lippes loop and the Margulies spiral were being systematically evaluated by the Population Council's statistical program, whereas independently developed models such as the Saf-T-Coil and the Dalkon Shield were not. The council may have welcomed individual IUD inventors as a sign of overall acceptance of the method. Untested devices, however, undercut the organization's effort to appraise the contraceptive method through a systematic large-scale study.[37] Council members were particularly unimpressed with the Saf-T-Coil, finding the company representative "abysmally ignorant of IUDs" and being "very vague" about the device's clinical performance.[38] Yet IUDs were classified as therapeutic devices, and therefore unregulated by the FDA, so the manufacturer was able to advertise the Saf-T-Coil in major medical journals, claiming that the device was safe and effective. A 1969 Saf-T-Coil advertisement, for instance, shows a large headline reading, "Off the pill . . . now what?" This message was printed along with phrases such as "the device of first choice" and "for almost every patient."[39] Elaborate advertisements for the Dalkon Shield were also placed in medical journals with data that exaggerated its effectiveness.[40]

Impending Infections

During these early years, the Population Council was mainly focused on the efficacy of the device; safety quickly became a secondary consideration. Researchers were well aware that most American doctors stayed away from intrauterine contraception for fear of infection, a serious problem experienced with European devices of the 1920s and 1930s and pessaries of the nineteenth century.[41] Thus, in his opening remark at the first international conference sponsored by the council in 1962, chairman Alan Guttmacher announced that their objective was to "find out scientifically, honestly, and in depth" whether the IUD was a good contraceptive method. He declared that if anyone "[felt] that its use is hazardous or ineffective," then "we must be frank in our appraisal."[42] Discussions during the conference, however, did not lead to a cautionary assessment. Most of the forty-eight conference participants already held a positive view of IUDs. They believed in the need for population control and, keen on offering their device as a solution, were reluctant to engage with the possibility that the device could pose health risks to individual users. Many presenters reported having seen some complications, but they almost always underplayed their seriousness, claiming that the infections they observed in their patients were rare and had been controlled with antibiotics.[43] Some physicians asserted that women were unnecessarily frightened, insinuated that their pain must be psychologically induced, and complained that they were being forced to remove IUDs at their patients' requests.[44]

Don Jessen of the Chicago Wesley Memorial Hospital was the only physician to assert that the IUD was not suitable for the indigent population. Based on his own experience with 121 patients (109 of whom were "negro"), as well as on the assumption that the incidence of inadequate hygiene and pelvic infection was higher among the poor, Jessen concluded, "I would not recommend this method unless close medical supervision is possible, and 100 percent follow-up is certain. . . . In short, this method, as I used it, is unsuited for general use as a contraceptive."[45] His dissenting voice, however, was drowned out by the overwhelming approval for the device by others at the conference who seemed to support Christopher Tietze's position that "the risks to life and health, inherent in the use of intra-uterine pessaries, appear to have been greatly exaggerated. The risks are certainly much smaller now than they were in the years around the 1930s."[46]

The overall tendency to underplay any health risks continued during the second Population Council conference in 1964. One researcher explained, "The inflammatory changes which occur with the plastic device are so little different from the inflammatory changes which occur normally in menstrual cycles," and then declared, "We should not let anxiety inhibit our enthusiasm for these devices, which are an enormous contribution to fertility control."[47] Viewing individual patient screening for contraindication to be counterproductive to the goal of accomplishing IUD insertions by large numbers, developers pushed aside prophylactic gynecology with their eagerness to apply this method to the masses. As a result, they ignored the cautionary lessons from the past and dismissed the skeptics.

A few years after IUDs became commercialized, an opportunity presented itself to investigate the safety of their use: three deaths from overwhelming infection in association with IUD use were reported in May 1967 to the FDA's Advisory Committee on Obstetrics and Gynecology. The committee responded by sending a survey to 8,500 doctors.[48] Among the 6,500 gynecologists who replied, there were ten deaths and 561 cases of critical infections or perforations associated with IUDs. Roger Scott, who headed the survey for the FDA, was sufficiently alarmed and tried to warn his colleagues, stating, "Complications from the use of IUDs may provide a fertile field for malpractice suits."[49] The advisory committee, however, judged that mortality, pelvic inflammatory disease, and perforation cases were negligible and failed in its 1968 FDA report to convey the sense of urgency that Scott had put forth.[50]

It is hardly surprising that the medical community and the FDA reacted so slowly when we examine the turn of events involving the IUD and oral contraceptives side by side. Although medical journals were writing cautionary appraisals of the pill, researchers did not begin to seriously examine its health effects until 1964, seven years after the FDA had approved the medication for gynecological treatment. Historian Elizabeth Watkins illustrates how enthusiasm and optimism regarding the pill permeated the media and the pharmaceutical industry, as well as physicians and women, delaying the serious questioning of its potential risks. During the first half of the 1960s, the pill's side effects such as headaches and nausea were believed to be treatable with other medications. Watkins points out that this was an era when the public still tended to trust in technological solutions to all problems, a mentality that also helped trivialize the pill's possible ill effects. Eventually by the late 1960s, the media moved away from its prior idealization of the pill and started to publish more critical articles. But in its 1969 report on oral contraceptives, the FDA still assured its safety. It was not until 1970, when the health effects of the pill were questioned in a congressional hearing and feminist activists voiced their concerns, that the FDA finally responded by requiring pharmaceutical companies to disclose known risks to patients.[51]

Ironically, the pill controversy did not prompt people to question the safety of the IUD; rather it created an opportunity for the devices to advance as an alternative birth control method. As studies began to connect dangerous blood clots to pill use, articles expressing doubts about the drug appeared in numerous popular magazines and newspapers. An increasing number of women quit using the pill, citing physical problems they had personally experienced or concerns over reports of adverse health effects.[52] In a Planned Parenthood Clinic in Detroit, requests for IUDs doubled over a month in 1970 as a result of patients who were discontinuing the pill. The New York City clinic also reported that one-fifth of oral contraceptive users had switched to the IUD or a diaphragm.[53] As women's demand grew for IUDs, a doctor in Boston reportedly had to install a second telephone to handle the volume of calls he received from women.[54]

Amid the controversy over the pill, IUD developers remained generally enthusiastic and optimistic about the device's potential as a technological solution to population control (if perhaps also overly confident that antibiotics would eliminate all serious health problems). Hugh Davis in fact seized this opportunity to promote his "modern" IUD while testifying as a Johns Hopkins University expert about the risks of the pill.[55] Condemning the hormonal method, Davis stated during an evening newscast, "Never in history have so many individuals taken such potent drugs with so little information as to actual potential hazards."[56] Regrettably, within several months, his hazardous shield device started being inserted into millions of women without sufficient information about its dangers.

Capitalizing on the doubts over the pill, Hugh Davis and A. H. Robins recruited women to use the Dalkon Shield. Since direct marketing of prescription pharmaceutical products was prohibited at the time, A. H. Robins appealed directly to consumers by arranging for articles that referred favorably to the Dalkon Shield in women's magazines.[57] Well-meaning feminist health advocates fell prey to the shield promotion and endorsed it. Barbara Seaman, a strong feminist critic of the health hazards of the pill, had the foreword to her popular book, *The Doctor's Case against the Pill*, written by Hugh Davis; she also discussed the shield positively in the book.[58] The 1973 edition of Boston Women's Health Collective's *Our Bodies Our Selves* also referred to IUDs in reassuring terms, even mentioning the shield by name.[59]

With impeccably tragic timing, the introduction of the Dalkon Shield coincided with the founding of campus health centers that emerged during the early 1970s with assistance from the Planned Parenthood World Population at the requests of American college students who were feeling the need for such services on campus.[60] Although the proportion of IUD use on campus was small compared to other methods, some young women did receive the Dalkon Shield through college health centers. The variety of outlets, including clinics, private physicians, and campus health centers, combined with the aggressive marketing of the Dalkon Shield, resulted in IUD insertions in young American women from all backgrounds.

Sterilizing injuries associated with IUDs in the United States crossed racial and class boundaries. By 1970, IUD adoption rates among women using contraception were similar between college-educated white women

(8.4 percent) and black women without a high school education (9.3 percent).[61] While many women had the IUD prescribed by providers who advocated fertility limitation for underprivileged women, testimonies indicate that some middle-class women chose the device based on what they had learned through the popular media and from their health care providers. One Dalkon Shield victim recounts, "I gained a lot of weight on [the pill]. My body became swollen, and I felt like an elephant."[62] When she decided to go off the pill, she requested the Dalkon Shield at the university health service based on the information it had provided her. The contraceptive choice she made led to a severe and prolonged pelvic infection, resulting in a surgery that left her sterile at the age of twenty-five.

Women who requested the IUD often expressed a strong desire to avoid getting pregnant as well as the burden of the pill's side effects as the reason for their choice. Because abortion was still illegal, many women who requested the IUD did so despite having to endure a different but equally terrible set of side effects, not because the method was ideal but because there were no other acceptable options. The unavailability of reliable contraceptive methods formed the basis for the "choices" that American women made in the 1960s and 1970s. And these were decisions they made without the knowledge of the infection rates and the fact that risks to women's health were largely overlooked in formal scientific studies of both the pill and IUD. Doctors, who were generally unaware of or unconcerned about potential dangers of these modern contraceptives, often dismissed women's complaints about severe pain and bleeding as psychological and called them "normal" side effects. The result was delayed treatment until the infections had irreversibly damaged the patients' reproductive organs.[63]

Without exonerating A. H. Robins for its greed and neglect, these historically specific situations of the United States—women's desire for better contraceptives, doctors' dismissive attitudes toward women's ailments, and the FDA's lack of regulatory power—all contributed to the large number of women who were harmed by the early distributions of the IUD. More important, the enthusiasm toward mass insertion had enticed its developers to consider the contraceptive method inherently safe for everyone. The debacle over the Dalkon Shield's safety finally reversed this situation. Not only were health risks studied more carefully, but the problems with the shield resulted in redefining who the ideal user was. Before I turn to that story, however, I recount the Population Council's involvement in the development of copper-bearing IUDs, which took place as the Dalkon Shield fallout was unraveling.

Copper-Bearing Devices and the Nullip IUD

Reviewing the Population Council's work on the development of copper-bearing devices here provides an important context for later discussion of how IUD supporters responded to the Dalkon Shield crisis. It also shows how the most globally prevalent IUD (and the model I received in 2002) originated. The development of copper-bearing devices overlapped with the emergence of "nullip" IUDs, or models for nulliparous women (those who had not previously borne children). Hence it is appropriate to discuss them together. Furthermore, the developers' interest in the nullips as attractive users accentuates the irony in their later definition of mothers as the only safe users.

Inventing the Copper T

The many different types of plastic IUDs devised during the 1960s did not result in one perfect device that would simultaneously lower the rates of pregnancy and side effects. Bulky models designed to fill up the uterus to achieve a low pregnancy rate, in particular, tended to cause more bleeding and cramping than other models, which led to an unacceptably high rate of removals. By the late 1960s, the Population Council was seeking ways to reduce the side effects in order to improve the rate of acceptance and retention of IUDs. The efforts of two council-affiliated scientists were aimed at this goal. Howard Tatum reversed the design concept that aimed at achieving the most coverage of the uterine cavity and went small. His T-shaped device reduced the undesirable symptoms, but its pregnancy rate, at 18 percent, was too high. Around the same time, Jaime Zipper discovered the antifertility effect of copper embedded in the uteruses of rodents.[64] The council subsequently combined the two innovations and tested a T-shaped device with a copper wire wound around it. The copper T IUD turned out to be a success, yielding a pregnancy rate of 1 percent after a twelve-month trial ending in 1970.[65]

As Anni Dugdale points out, the Population Council had a number of motives for pursuing the development of a copper-bearing IUD. It had just acquired a new laboratory facility. Studying the copper-bearing device provided the organization with an attractive project that would combine its new biomedical research capability with applied research and clinical testing. The organization was also in need of a new device for India, where its initial effort to disseminate IUDs had failed. The IUD campaigns in India had quickly met resistance from women who removed their devices on their own and told others not to accept one. The Population Council believed that the program was unsuccessful because of administrative shortfalls. But local family planning clinics turned away from IUDs, claiming that the devices did not suit local conditions. Indian clinicians stipulated that a new device with better acceptability, namely one that did not have the troublesome side effect of heavy bleeding, be provided before they would once again try adopting this contraceptive method. The copper T thus "provided hope for a new opportunity to introduce intrauterine devices into the Indian context."[66] In short, the copper-bearing IUD was initially conceived as an improved and more scientific device for limiting the fertility of the global South.

Teen Pregnancy and the Nullip IUD

When researchers started experimenting with the plastic IUDs in the early 1960s, they were ambivalent about their use in nulliparous women, whom they viewed as anatomically different from women who had given birth. They occasionally created smaller experimental models for nulliparous women, but were divided on how well this group tolerated the insertion procedure and side effects. Expulsion rates also appeared to be unacceptably high in this population.[67] But IUD developers were not too worried about childless women because limiting the reproductive capacities of women with multiple children was considered more critical to the goal of curbing population growth. Hence, clinical testing focused mostly on women who had children; 97 percent of the participants of the five-year large-scale trial that lasted from 1963 to 1968 were women who had children.[68] Then the new copper T trial found that women with no children retained this device better than they did the older plastic ones. The timing of this finding coincided with the rise of the American public's interest in teen pregnancies.

In the late 1960s, the focus of U.S. domestic birth control politics started to steer away from the excess fertility of the indigent and toward the problem of teen pregnancy. Amid the civil rights and women's movements and the protest against the Vietnam War, adolescent pregnancy had become another source of anxiety over social upheaval. In Constance Nathanson's view, increased pregnancies in white middle-class teenagers symbolized the fears of dominant social groups that society as they knew it was disintegrating.[69] Adolescent sexuality, which until then had been a local problem of families, schools, and health care providers, was thus elevated to a national problem. Fortunately for family planning advocates, concerns over teen pregnancy allowed them to mobilize public sentiment to garner more support for their programs during a time when the Nixon administration was cutting welfare dollars. Planned Parenthood–assisted college campus reproductive health centers emerged against this social and political background. As Dugdale argues, public interest in a contraceptive method for young women, combined with the positive test results of nulliparous women, led the Population Council to position copper-bearing devices potentially appropriate for women who had not borne children.[70]

Due in part to the 1971 reclassification of copper-bearing devices as a drug that required FDA premarketing testing approval, the council's copper T device was not released in the United States until 1976. Meanwhile other IUD developers devised nullip models independently and marketed them as suitable for young women. One was a smaller version of the Dalkon Shield, which A. H. Robins marketed without sufficient testing.[71] The shield indeed became the contraceptive method of choice for two gynecologists serving "high-risk young girls" at the Cincinnati Adolescent Clinic during the 1970s. They wrote that the shield, with its lower expulsion rate, was ideal for their patients, whom they regarded as "a population group that keeps appointments poorly and moves frequently" and had "a 30 percent patient failure rate with the pills."[72] Just as the representation of women of the global South as unmotivated supported the need for IUDs, assumptions about what were referred to as high-risk and unreliable young women reaffirmed the benefit of the long-term effectiveness of the device in controlling problematic fertility in subpopulations of the global North.

In 1974 G. D. Searle became the first company to market a copper-bearing device in the United States.[73] Its Copper-7 was shaped like the number seven and came with a slimmer inserter, features that were considered more suitable for the smaller uteruses and cervical openings of young and nulliparous women. Remarkably, the Copper-7 managed to capture this market right after the Dalkon Shield was withdrawn and physicians were becoming more cautious with IUD insertions. Targeted promotion helped open up the new market for the slighter Copper-7, which was advertised as a device that avoided the symptoms of cramping and bleeding that few young women were able to tolerate. Searle made 40 percent of its sales of copper-bearing devices to nulliparous women and 75 percent to women younger than twenty-five years old.[74] Young women, then, became ideal IUD users in two ways during the 1970s: as a new site of problematic pregnancies in the public arena and as a new market segment. These new users emerged in tandem with the development of smaller copper-bearing IUDs in conjunction with alternative biopolitical scripts for this contraceptive method.

In fact, the idea of a nullip IUD was relatively short-lived. When Gyno-Pharma became the new American distributor of the copper T in 1988, it labeled young childless women as inappropriate users, arguing that studies had shown this group to be more prone to pelvic inflammatory diseases. This transition occurred in the context of IUD supporters' efforts to save the contraceptive method from the Dalkon Shield fallout. Researchers who had invested funds, energy, and hope in advancing IUDs as a superior family planning method quickly responded to the public questioning of the safety of the IUD and worked to restore its reputation.

Rehabilitating the IUD: The Co-Configuration of the "Safe" Technology and Body

When Russel Thomsen publicly reproved gynecologists who experimented with IUDs in 1973, copper T development was under way with positive indications.[75] Within two weeks of the Thomsen hearing, three IUD researchers testified for the Population Council before the House Committee on Government Operations. Daniel Mishell Jr., Sheldon Segal, and Christopher Tietze expressed support for Thomsen's call for FDA regulations of the contraceptive method; they also presented an expert's recommendation for a standard for evaluating the efficacy and safety of different IUDs. Most important, they expressed their confidence in the integrity of the IUD itself as a contraceptive method and emphasized that the Population Council had conducted extensive studies through its large-scale multisite clinical trial program, which verified the adequacy of the most widely used models.[76] From this 1973 testimony through the 1988 reintroduction of the copper T to the American market, researchers affiliated with the Population Council and independent researchers took active roles in rehabilitating the IUD as a safe and acceptable contraceptive method. Their efforts involved several strategies, including placing the blame on the Dalkon Shield device, locating any risk of using the device in users' sexual behavior, and redefining the ideal user. Through these research activities and new discourse, an alternative biopolitical script was configured for the contraceptive method: one that deemed mothers as the safe subjects and required careful screening and disciplining of prospective users.

Isolating the Dalkon Shield

Howard Tatum of the Biomedical Division of the Population Council conducted studies that arguably had the most impact on isolating the Dalkon Shield as a uniquely dangerous device.[77] Most IUDs today have a tail: a thread that extends from within the uterus, through the cervical opening, and into the vagina so that the device can be easily located and removed. Tatum dipped one end of the tail taken from various IUDs in dye and showed that only the tail of the Dalkon Shield, which was made of multiple fibers encased in a sheath as opposed to a single-filament fiber like all other IUDs, allowed the dye to flow from one end to the other. Tatum also observed that many of the tails of Dalkon Shields that had been removed from patients had breaks in them below the knot that resided inside the uterus, which indicated that infectious material could travel from the unsterile vagina into a normally sterile uterus via the tail. This observation suggested that the multifilament tail of the Dalkon Shield might have served as a wick, drawing bacteria up from the vagina into the uterine cavity. Furthermore, Tatum noticed that when a woman became pregnant with the shield, the tail, which most likely harbored bacteria from the vagina between the filaments, usually retracted into the enlarging uterus after about ten weeks. This explained why the most severe infections and septic abortions in Dalkon Shield users occurred in the second trimester of pregnancy. Tatum presented his findings at the congressional hearing in August 1974, and published his findings in the *Journal of the American Medical Association* the following year.[78]

Daniel Mishell continued to offer his support after making an appearance in front of the Congress. The following year, he published an article in *Family Planning Perspectives*, laying out study results that indicated that

the Dalkon Shield was especially dangerous.[79] Frederick Clarke, vice president and medical director of the A. H. Robins Company, tried to discount
Mishell's conclusion, arguing in a dissenting letter to the editor that it was
plausible that all IUDs were responsible for a higher incidence of pelvic
inflammatory disease (PID). But Mishell quickly responded with a rebut-
tal, concluding that the shield was more prone to perforating the uterus
and the multifilament tail could explain the increased numbers of fatal
and nonfatal cases of sepsis (the presence of microorganisms in the uterine
environment) in shield users.[80]

Today the wicking tail theory is generally accepted by the medical community as the explanation for the high incidence of Dalkon Shield deaths
and injuries.[81] Eliminating the shield certainly appears to have improved
the overall safety of intrauterine contraception. But it also secured a new
status for the copper T as a physically different, better, and safer device.[82]
This was the first phase of the construction of a "safe technology." Holding certain IUD users responsible for their own injuries also facilitated this
process.

Locating Risk in Sexual Behavior

The category of users I call "risky and promiscuous" emerged from epidemiological studies during the 1980s aimed at investigating the relationship
between IUD use and adverse health effects. The 1981 Women's Health
Study looked at risk factors for PID, including IUDs. Overall, the highest
risk factor among women without prior PID history was having more than
one sexual partner, which raised the risk of PID by 2.6 times. Having sexual
intercourse more than five times a week and being younger than twenty-
five raised the risk by 1.9 times, being an African American raised it by 1.8
times, and using an IUD by 1.6 times, which led the authors to conclude
that IUD use substantially increased the risk of hospitalization with a first
episode of PID. The data, however, showed that women with multiple sexual partners using an IUD had a lower relative risk of hospitalization with
PID compared to nonusers than did IUD users with a single sexual partner
compared to nonusers. In other words, this particular set of data did not
suggest that IUD users with multiple sexual partners were at higher risk of
becoming infected with a severe case of PID than users with only one partner. Nonetheless, the authors warned that IUD use might have contributed
to the highest rate of hospitalization with PID in women who have multiple

sexual partners, therefore suggesting that the two risk factors might have a compounding effect.[83]

The number of sexual partners as a risk factor was examined in another study published a few years later. This time, the researchers found that when copper IUD users had multiple sexual partners, their risk of developing PID was elevated by 2.8 times; for users of other types of IUDs, the risk increased by 4.2 times. They also discovered that users who reported having only one sexual partner had no increased risk of tubal infertility associated with IUD use. The authors maintained that they did not want to overemphasize the importance of number of sexual partners as a contributing factor. Nonetheless, the report left an impression that the user's sexual activity could be a risk factor.[84]

Finally, in 1988, a group of researchers who reanalyzed the data from the Women's Health Study by marital status suggested that the sexual activities of both the IUD user and her partner factored into PID risk. They found that an IUD user who was married or cohabiting had a negligible increase of risk of PID compared to non-IUD users. Simultaneously they found that even if an IUD user reported having only one recent sexual partner, her risk of PID increased by 1.8 times and 2.6 times if the woman was not currently married or not cohabiting. After a disclaimer statement that they had no evidence to back up their hypothesis, the authors speculated that sexually transmitted pathogens might account for the increased cases of PID and that promiscuous sexual activity by the women or their sexual partners, or both partners, might be the source of increased cases of the disease in these women. The authors conjectured that married or cohabiting IUD users were most likely in mutually monogamous relationships, which decreased the risk of contracting an infectious disease. They also insinuated that women who reported having only one recent sexual partner but were neither married nor cohabiting were at increased risk of PID because their partners were not monogamous.[85]

Through selective reading of epidemiological data, these medical texts neatly localized IUD risks to promiscuous sexual behavior of the users and their partners. Although the authors carefully worded their findings as hypotheses or just one possible factor, other researchers interpreted the studies as showing that sexual promiscuity increased the health risks associated with IUD use as a plausible explanation. This association, which relocated the fault of injuries to the users' lifestyle, allowed researchers to presume it was not the IUD that posed a risk to women but that some women engaged in sexual behavior that made them too risky for the IUD.

These risky and promiscuous users who emerged from the medical discourse were inevitably judged against cultural ideals of sexual morality. Asking the plaintiffs detailed questions about their sexual activities became one of the dirty tricks that the defense lawyers of A. H. Robins used in litigation over the Dalkon Shield. Although such questions did not necessarily lead in court to faulting the women for contracting PID, this spiteful, intimidating tactic might have caused some women who considered suing for Dalkon Shield–related injuries not to do so.[86]

Excluding Childless Women

Being nulliparous was also added to the profile of users considered risky after the Dalkon Shield catastrophe. What made the shield fallout particularly tragic was that it left many young women who had never had children sterile from the infections they had suffered. A. H. Robins had started marketing the nullip model in late 1970 without adequate safety or efficacy studies.[87] After Hughs announced that his three-year study had yielded favorable results, the sales of the nullip model rose to 883,500 in 1972. Soon after, individual studies started reporting that the nullip shield was not living up to its advertisements: the pregnancy rate and the rate of removal due to pain, bleeding, and infection were much higher than anticipated. Nevertheless, A. H. Robins never appropriately warned practitioners that the product might not perform as effectively as advertised. Consequently thousands of young, childless American women were injured and sterilized.[88]

One question that arises is whether using other IUDs put nulliparous women at a higher risk of PID and tubal infertility, and, if so, whether they should be prohibited from using the method. Studies during the 1970s and 1980s produced confusing results and mixed responses. One 1978 review of epidemiological studies suggested that a higher risk of PID was found among younger nulliparous women using IUDs compared to nonusers.[89] Such a finding was enough to prompt Ortho Pharmaceuticals to add to its Lippes loop product label for both physicians and patients that the risk of tubal infertility "appears to be greatest for nulliparous women and those exposed to multiple sex partners."[90] Searle did not use similar labeling and later was accused of not providing such information explicitly. The company lost a multiple-million-dollar suit in which it was also charged with misrepresenting the Copper-7 as ideal for women without children despite knowing that the device's stem might be too long for the uterus of a typical nulliparous woman.[91]

When GynoPharma reintroduced the copper T in the United States in 1988 with the help of the Population Council, IUD advocates had witnessed Searle's legal defeat. Considering the personal and social implications of a nulliparous woman's loss of fertility, the device was released as a contraceptive method for mothers only. An overall sense of taboo among the researchers against inserting IUDs in women without children permeated at the time. This is reflected in the 1988 issue of *Population Reports* published by the Population Information Program at the Johns Hopkins University, which announced that the IUD should not be the first choice of contraception for a woman who has no children yet but eventually wants them.[92] *Population Reports* was designed to provide family planning programs overseas with up-to-date information on important developments in the field. This suggests that IUD experts in the late 1980s refrained from promoting IUDs to nulliparous women regardless of their geographical location.

Researchers, however, soon recognized that studies published before or during the 1980s still included Dalkon Shield users in their data, which tended to inflate the overall rate of health risk.[93] Some studies also did not account for patients' previous history of PID or the possibility that an existing infection was transmitted into the uterus at the time of IUD insertion. Accordingly, the international family planning community reversed the recommendation against prescribing IUDs to nulliparous women after several years, and the 1995 issue of *Population Reports* no longer proscribed the IUD for these women. It instead cited the World Health Organization (WHO) scientific working group's newly developed eligibility criteria for copper IUDs, which put childless women into a category of users for whom "advantages generally outweigh theoretical or proven disadvantages." The working group concluded that "copper-bearing IUDs generally can be provided without restriction."[94] The international standards were thus loosened at the same time that the copper T continued to be strictly limited to women with children in the United States.

This double standard stems from social considerations. Besides the discomfort that tends to be more intense in a smaller uterus and the slightly

higher expulsion rate, there is no clear biological indication that nulliparous uteruses are somehow more prone to infection associated with IUD
use. Being childless is a social argument against IUD use rather than a
medical one. Some French physicians admitted not prescribing IUDs to
childless women, not because these women were thought to have a higher
risk of infection and subsequent sterility, but rather because should they
sustain injury, the "consequences [were] considered more serious for this
group."[95]

In the United States, a group of physicians studying the relationship between tubal infertility and IUD use observed that few women with multiple
children consulted a physician for infertility. They concluded their 1985 article in the *New England Journal of Medicine* by reasoning that copper-bearing
devices are adequate for women who already have more than one child
because "multiparous women are unlikely to consult a fertility specialist
and hence least likely to regret the decision to use an IUD."[96] Implicit in
this conclusion is that a woman who becomes infertile after having borne
children is less likely to be disturbed by this unfortunate event should it
befall her. These researchers subtly defined multiparous women as "safer"
from regret and less prone to litigation and nulliparous women as "riskier"
IUD users from a social point of view.

With these findings and ideas in mind, the new brand name for
the copper T device, ParaGard, was chosen to suggest to doctors that
the product was appropriate for a parous woman (one who has given
birth).[97] In the 1988 market reintroduction video aimed at physicians,
gynecologist Dr. William J. Ledger of New York offered assurances that
researchers had identified the factors that had contributed to injuries
associated with IUD use in the past. He maintained that the new device was an ideal contraceptive for many women, particularly since safer
and more effective approaches to clinical use had been developed. He
emphasized that IUDs had unfortunately been aggressively promoted
to "women who would have been a bad selection" or "inappropriate
users," and he insisted that with proper patient screening, the device
was safe.[98] GynoPharma then promoted its product in medical journals
with an advertisement featuring a mother, father, and two young children (a boy and a girl), indicating clearly that a ParaGard user should
be a married woman with children who has completed her reproductive
goals (figure 3.1).[99]

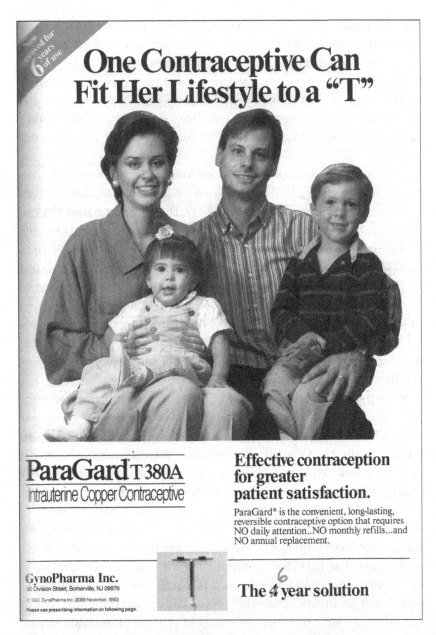

Figure 3.1
This advertisement depicts the ideal user of ParaGard (copper T IUD) as a married mother with two children. (GynoPharma, *Obstetrics and Gynecology*, 1991)

Safeguarding with Informed Consent

ParaGard also came with "the most informative consumer information leaflet ever released," preempting allegations of misinformation that led G. D. Searle to its downfall in court.[100] GynoPharma and the Population Council understood that assuring American physicians that the new device was safe and efficacious when inserted into an "appropriate" body would not be sufficient to appease their fears. Before medical professionals would start supplying IUDs again to their patients, they would have to feel protected from malpractice suits. The ParaGard-launching symposium therefore featured an energetic lawyer, Nancy Ledy Gurren, who made a presentation on how to use informed consent as the "physician's ultimate defense." She urged physicians to guard themselves with documentation as protection against being sued.[101]

Informed consent was not undertaken for contraceptive products when the IUD first hit the American market in the 1960s. It was put into practice only in 1970, after women's health activists demanded full disclosure of known risks associated with pill use and the FDA ordered manufacturers to include inserts for patients describing these risks in every package of birth control pills.[102] The feminists' aim was to enable women to make informed decisions about birth control, which was in line with the women's health movement of the time that tried to empower women with knowledge and give them control over their bodies.[103] Relinquishing their absolute authority and allowing patients to have information was threatening to health providers, however, and therefore pharmaceutical companies and most physicians at the time vehemently resisted the package labeling inserts. A few doctors nevertheless favored the insert, arguing that it would "serve as a protection for the doctor."[104] In fact, the American Medical Association counseled physicians to give their patients information about the advantages and disadvantages of the pill and other methods of birth control "to protect themselves against possible malpractice suits."[105] The original feminist intention of informed consent was to preserve the moral right of the patient to make educated decisions about health care. But the idea that the practice of informed consent serves to protect doctors also existed from the very beginning. Not surprisingly, when the copper T was reintroduced to American physicians, considerable emphasis was placed on the role of informed consent as a means to safeguard health practitioners.

Fourteen years later, informed consent indeed helped protect an IUD manufacturer and health care provider in the 2002 case of *Snyder* v. *Ortho-McNeil Pharmaceuticals*. The Snyders, a couple in California, filed a personal injury complaint against Ortho-McNeil Pharmaceuticals alleging that its copper T IUD failed to prevent pregnancy; moreover, it had become embedded in Mrs. Snyder's uterus and perforated her uterine wall. The suit also alleged medical malpractice against the nurse-midwife who inserted the IUD in the client in May 1999.

According to court records, Mrs. Snyder signed the informed consent form acknowledging that she had read the brochure for patients in its entirety and that her health care provider had answered all of her questions about the risks and benefits associated with the IUD. The Snyders asserted product liability under the consumer expectation test; that is, they claimed the product failed to perform as safely as an ordinary consumer would expect when used in an intended or reasonably foreseeable manner. Although the IUD did not prevent pregnancy and did perforate the uterus, the panel ruled that the Snyders could not rely on those facts because they had been adequately warned by the health care provider and the informed consent form included in the IUD package that both adverse effects could happen. The Snyders' negligence claim against the nurse-midwife was also dismissed because the appeals court judged that there was no evidence that she had breached the ordinary standard of care or failed to show the reasonable degree of skill, knowledge, and care ordinarily possessed by members of the profession under similar circumstances.[106]

Like Mrs. Snyder, a woman who receives an IUD today is given a patient information booklet written in small print and a form to sign stating that she has read and understood the information and that all questions have been answered. As the Snyders' case exemplifies, however, the informed consent practice does not necessarily protect the woman from health risks; instead it makes her conform to the norms of the capital market, requiring her to be the willing and legally (but not necessarily physically) safe consumer of a product.

The Co-Configuration of Technology and Body
To summarize, restoring the IUD as a contraceptive method in the United States required (1) isolating the Dalkon Shield as a uniquely dangerous model; (2) locating risk factors in the user's sexual behavior as the source

of sexually transmitted diseases that could cause pelvic inflammatory disease leading to infertility; (3) identifying married mothers or women in a mutually monogamous relationship as ideal safe users, while eliminating nulliparous, young, and promiscuous women as posing risks of infections as well as malpractice suits; and (4) preempting IUD recipients' litigious behaviors through the practice of informed consent. The new ideal IUD user, an older married mother who is not interested in continued fertility, was co-configured with the new safe technology through this process. She closely resembled the person that I represented to my Planned Parenthood doctor. I embodied the socially constructed safe IUD user.[107]

By redefining the appropriate user, developers were able to argue that this technology was inherently safe and that IUDs had been inserted in the wrong women in the past. A safe technology, then, was renegotiated in conjunction with a safe body through material and discursive rearrangements in the post–Dalkon Shield era of the history of the IUD. The safe body was also a carefully disciplined body that adhered to health screening, sexual monogamy, and informed consent. An ironic situation ensued whereby the more privileged consumer, who is often presumed to have more reproductive freedom, became subjected to closer scrutiny over her choice of contraception. This mode of governance was primarily developed for Western consumers, whose injuries generated public outcry and damaged corporate image and profitability. A series of epidemiological studies that distinguished bodies viewed as safe from those considered risky played a significant role in formulating this new biopolitical script. The co-constitutive relationship between science and biopower is strongly represented in this case.

From the Masses to the Moms and Back to the Nullips

IUD distribution in the United States could have simply ended when pharmaceutical companies withdrew their products in the mid-1980s after facing hundreds of lawsuits and the rising cost of liability insurance. Yet the Population Council reintroduced the copper T device to the American market with the premise of fulfilling the contraceptive needs of American women. William Ledger, narrating the ParaGard promotional video in 1988, underscored that the introduction of IUDs during the 1960s as an alternative to the pill was "a marvelous event," and that the device was "a much needed contraceptive by American women."[108] Yet it was somewhat unrealistic to expect that a small one-product company like GynoPharma could build a wide distribution network. While worldwide IUD users expanded from 85 million to 106 million and the number of IUDs in developing countries (excluding China) grew from 14.4 million to 25.6 million between 1987 and 1995, the number of North American users plummeted from approximately 1.8 million users to 650,000.[109] Who, then, gained from bringing the device back to the United States?

When pharmaceutical companies stopped selling IUDs in the United States in 1986, national and international health and family planning organizations protested. The family planning community recognized that the first to be affected were American women, 2.2 million of whom were using the IUD in 1982. The Planned Parenthood Federation of America reaffirmed its support of IUDs by announcing that they were reliable forms of reversible contraception. The American Health Association called for "immediate measures to bring back . . . the FDA approved copper-bearing IUDs."[110] All lamented the peculiar American legal climate that made the contraceptive method economically unviable.

But the withdrawal of IUD products in the United States also had "ramifications that extend far beyond the domestic market."[111] Donor agencies such as the United States Agency for International Development (USAID), International Planned Parenthood Federation, United Nations Fund for Population Activities, Family Planning International Assistance, the Pathfinder Fund, and the WHO were still providing IUDs on request to governments and private voluntary family planning agencies in the global South.[112] Some became worried that the pharmaceutical companies' actions would be misunderstood as taken in response to medical problems associated with the device and that "contraceptive providers and potential acceptors outside the United States [would] reject IUDs out of mistaken fears that they may be unsafe."[113]

Others fretted not so much that the availability of IUDs for use in overseas family planning programs would be severely affected, but that "political implications" would prove to be "extremely serious."[114] According to a family planning supporter, a Venezuelan newspaper had reported that companies had withdrawn IUDs from the U.S. market because of serious health risks to women and insinuated that unsafe devices were being dumped on women in the global South. A. H. Robins had in fact been accused of dumping the shields overseas about a decade earlier when they sold them at a large discount to USAID and the agency dispensed them after domestic sales were discontinued. IUD advocates were concerned that Western donors and the U.S. government might be accused of wrongdoing if they continued to distribute a contraceptive method that was no longer being sold to American women.[115]

In this situation, reintroducing IUDs to the U.S. market was an effective way to signal to the rest of the world that the contraceptive method was indeed considered safe for everyone.[116] Although IUD distribution overseas would probably not have totally collapsed and even if the 1988 ParaGard reintroduction had had only a small impact on improving contraceptive choice for American women, its availability in the United States helped appease any doubts about the device internationally. Enforcing a strict screening protocol to identify safe individuals for insertion in the United States tacitly protected the copper T from another fallout that might endanger its status as a marketable product. Thus on the one hand, the legitimacy of IUDs as a contraceptive was sustained by their reintroduction in the United States. On the other hand, American women regained limited access to IUDs because their developers wanted to sustain the reputation of this method to continue its distribution in family planning programs overseas. These negotiations transformed the IUD into a contraceptive for the masses as well as moms through quite disparate yet interlocking rationales.

For more than a decade after the WHO guidelines sanctioned copper T use in childless women, however, U.S. distributors continued to officially market their IUDs only to mothers. Hence, two types of scenarios of IUD insertions, or biopolitical scripts coexisted: one that excluded young, childless Western women and the other that targeted the masses, including women without children. Feminist scholars have critiqued how divergent risk assessments for contraceptives are applied to different subjects. Jessica van Kammen and Nelly Oudshoorn, for instance, compare risk models for male and female contraceptives over a period of thirty years and point out that risks for women are downplayed compared to risks for men.[117] Risk models for the masses and individual consumers are also often disparate. Health risks for women in the global North using a contraceptive method are often compared to the conditions of healthy, untreated women, which leads to the judgment that they are unacceptably high. The risk of infection for women in the global South is often compared to the risk of maternity and deemed as acceptable or less dangerous. Such an argument allows the WHO to prescribe IUDs to nulliparous women on account of the various benefits of avoiding pregnancy. [118]

As Adrienne Germain and Ruth Dixon-Muller point out, contraceptive distribution in the global South is too often justified based on the reasoning that the mortality risk from using contraception is smaller than the mortality risk of bearing a child. The maternity-based argument ignores the fact that depending on the circumstances, the side effects that affect women's daily lives or family members' opposition to contraception may pose graver risk to users than the remote risk of maternal death.[119] But more important, contraceptive risk calculations are often based on studies completed with patients in the global North. Therefore, health risks to low-income women in Southern countries with limited access to medical care may in fact be much higher. But when risk calculations are done, the numbers are assumed to be applicable to all women. While certain differences between women of the global North and South are emphasized in favor of family planning programs, other differences are obscured by presumed biological universality. IUD insertion protocols mirror this paradoxical discourse of sameness and divide between North and South, while the same epidemiological studies provide the basis for different arguments about who is an appropriate device recipient.

Significantly, Duramed Pharmaceuticals, the ParaGard distributor in the United States since 2006, overturned the insertion restriction against nulliparous women.[120] The company now markets the device to young childless women, citing a 2001 study that found copper IUD users to suffer no more infertility than nonusers as a justification for changing the user criteria for its product.[121] Although this modification is presented as a response to new scientific findings, it is also a crafty move to differentiate the ParGard from its rival product, Mirena, and expand the market base. Bayer Health-Care Pharmaceuticals, the distributor of the hormone-releasing IUD Mirena, which has been on the U.S. market since 2001, continues to hold that the product is primarily suitable for women who have children. Mirena's distributor explains that this designation is because the device has been mostly tested on parous women.[122] Through this conservative measure, the company hopes to avoid controversy. For both companies, how nulliparous women's bodies should be regulated is a question of balance between profitability and risk. The market now plays an additional significant role in the governance of women's bodies, to which we will turn again in chapter 5.

The safety of the modern IUD has no doubt improved greatly since its first introduction in the 1960s. Insertion techniques and procedures have been improved to prevent uterine perforation and bacterial infections. Faulty devices have been removed from the market. And healthcare providers are aware of potential complications and are thus more cautious in caring for their patients. Yet no contraceptives are 100 percent effective or free of health risks. Given this fact, it is difficult to say which approach better serves nulliparous women's interests. It may be more important to take cautious measures to limit the number of women who may experience adverse effects. However, if IUDs impose no greater health risk to young women than to older women, as the WHO claims, withholding them from the former and depriving them of a valuable contraceptive choice in the interest of protecting the company from a malpractice suit is unjust. In the end, however, whether a woman without children could have an IUD inserted is currently at the discretion of each provider in the United States. Doctors are the ultimate gatekeepers of women's choices.

Diffracting the Copper T: The Interlacing Biopolitical Subjects

This chapter has illustrated how the object I had inserted in my uterus in 2002 is a historical product composed of multiple development trajectories and discourses. The transformation the IUD made between the 1960s and today gave rise to various representations of appropriate and inappropriate users who are marked by their intersectional positions consisting of race, class, nationality, marital status, childbearing history, and presumed sexual behavior. Multiple biopolitical scripts also emerged as coproducts of implicated users, ranging from fertility restriction of racial minorities and lower-class women in the United States and prevention of white middle-class teen pregnancies to the preclusion of young, "promiscuous," and childless women from IUD insertions. Contradicting forms of governance, such as withholding IUDs from nulliparous women in the global North while advocating the device for the same category of people in the global South, existed simultaneously under disparate risk measurements. These multiple scripts, which are constantly under modification, constitute this technology.

This chapter also demonstrated the interrelationships between the constructions of users of the global North and the global South by tracing differently marked bodies genealogically. Those who were conceptualized as ideal American consumers of the IUD—beginning with racial minorities, who were subjects of negative eugenics, and teenagers, who "could not keep appointments to receive the pills," to married middle-class mothers, who have the "safest" bodies—were all generated through IUD researchers' efforts to develop and maintain a technology for the masses. Meanwhile the various biopolitical subjects circulating within the IUD discourse were differentially governed in keeping with the hierarchical positions women occupied in the global political economy. However, because female bodies are presumed to be biologically alike, differences among them were easily subsumed under the notion of universal technology. What this chapter has done is to diffract this contraceptive method through the shifting concept of risk and the global political economy of women's bodies. It has traced how the IUD has come to embody multiple meanings and how "my/our" contraceptive choice and a device that controls "their" fertility have been historically interconnected.

4 "IUDs Are Not Abortifacients": The Biopolitics of Contraceptive Mechanisms

Most scientific papers have agreed that in as many as 95 percent of the cases [the IUD] does not prevent fertilization. What it does do is prevent the implantation, at one week of life, of the tiny new human into the nutrient lining of the mother's womb. Because with that in place, this little boy or girl cannot implant, he or she dies and passes from the mother's body. So, even though your doctor may call an IUD a contraceptive, remember, it does not prevent fertilization. It does cause the death of the tiny new human at one week of life in a micro-abortion, and for this reason, few Christian women will allow one to be inserted into them.
—John Willke, M.D., Life Issues Institute

The characterization of the IUD as an abortifacient is a rhetorical move that has been advanced by antiabortion movement leaders and religiously inclined physicians. Discrediting contraceptive methods has been integral to the conservative political agenda in the United States, which gained a foothold with the New Right's rise to power during the 1980s. In the opening quote to this chapter, John Willke, a significant figure in the antiabortion movement, denounces the IUD mechanism of action in his role as the in-house medical specialist on the Life Issues Institute Web site.[1] He depicts the IUD as an object that causes a "micro-abortion" by preventing implantation, that is, the attachment of the fertilized egg to the maternal uterine wall. Scientists who have long been involved in IUD development disagree with his description. They explain that the IUD exerts its antifertility effect primarily by preventing fertilization and maintain that the device indisputably is a contraceptive method.

This controversy about abortion has been a source of dilemma for IUD developers since the early 1960s when they sought to revitalize the contraceptive method as a population control tool. Despite years of scientific research, the exact biological reactions induced by the device have never been identified. Over the years, developers have been especially careful to interpret and present the IUD's mechanism of action in a socially acceptable manner. The uncertainty of its functions, however, has given antiabortionists an opportunity to challenge the legitimacy of this contraceptive method. The dispute over the representation of the IUD's mechanism of action—Is it an antifertilization or an anti-implantation method?—is one of the battles that pro-contraceptive groups are forced to fight in the antichoice war waged by the religious and political Right. Although this debate has not been settled, IUD supporters' struggle to validate the antifertilization hypothesis has positioned them in a closer alliance with feminists who advocate broader access to reproductive health care and fertility control methods. Historical investigation of the representations of the IUD's mechanism of action reveals how conflicts and coalitions among divergent reproductive politics have shaped the scientific debate and contributed to the construction of a heterogeneous technological object.

This chapter traces the discourse of the IUD's mechanism of action from the 1960s to the present. First, I examine how developers of the device reconciled the method as a contraceptive and how they responded to pressures from the antiabortion camp over the years. Second, I situate the scientific debate within the broader political struggle and analyze the discursive construction of the IUD as an abortifacient. I argue that the perception that the device is an abortifacient is coconstructed with a representation of the "religious woman" and a patriarchal mode of governance over women's bodies. Finally, I elaborate how the war on choice has solidified a feminist/neo-Malthusian alliance and the support behind the notion of the IUD as a contraceptive choice. On the whole, this chapter shows how contesting views on the mechanism of the IUD were built in relationship to each other.

The IUD as Contraceptive

Eluding the Abortion Question: The 1960s to the 1970s
We begin in the 1960s, a time of both optimism and uncertainty surrounding the acceptability of the IUD's mechanism of action among the device's advocates. During the first international conference on the IUD hosted by the Population Council in 1962, Mary Calderone, a former medical director of the Planned Parenthood Federation of America, posed a crucial question:

"What is an abortion?" She proceeded to offer her opinion: "I think that this is an extremely important question that must be settled, because if it turns out that these intra-uterine devices operate as abortifacients, not only the Catholic church will be against them, but the Protestant churches as well. It is a philosophical as well as a physiological question, and the answer will depend on finding out just when and how the fertilized ovum is affected by these devices."[2] Lazar Margulies, recipient of the first IUD research grant from the council, conceded, "No one [has proven] . . . what happens every month to the women with devices *in utero*."[3] Margulies, however, believed that the foreign body caused the uterine wall to change in a way that prevented the implantation of the fertilized egg. Christopher Tietze, who took charge of the large-scale IUD clinical trial programs after this conference, offered an alternative view: the device prevents fertilization. He suggested that the lower rates of tubal pregnancies in IUD users compared to nonusers were an indication of much fewer incidents of fertilization.[4]

Following the conference, studies on the IUD's contraceptive mechanism were conducted with the intention of assisting the development of better devices with increased efficacy and decreased side effects and health risks. But researchers also knew that their study results had political ramifications in the context of the abortion question. They understood that the scientific representation of how the IUD works would influence its acceptance in both the United States and abroad.[5]

Meanwhile, in 1963, the U.S. Department of Health, Education and Welfare defined *abortion* as "all the measures which impair the viability of the zygote at any time between the instant of fertilization and the completion of labor," a definition that most antiabortionists still use today.[6] In the early 1960s, however, there was not a clear international consensus among physicians on whether abortion should be considered as interference at any time after the moment of fertilization or if it concerned terminating pregnancy only after implantation. Researchers and philanthropists who gathered for the second international IUD conference in 1964 clearly felt that there still was room left for maneuvering. Conference participants pondered the possibility of establishing a medical consensus that would equate the start of a pregnancy with implantation of the fertilized ovum. As Dr. Samuel Wishik from Pakistan reasoned, a medical definition potentially affected national policies: "In a Moslem country such as Pakistan, if it is considered that the IUD is an abortifacient, this obviously would have a bearing on national acceptance or rejection of the method. I think, therefore, the careful attention should be given to a definition of terms."[7] Wishik then proceeded to suggest defining *abortion* as taking away the embryo after it has implanted, arguing that since fertilized ova often fail to rest in the uterus for no obvious reason, implantation should be considered the beginning of pregnancy.

His peers were relatively confident that scientific reasoning would have authority over the theological and popular notions of what constitutes abortion. Christopher Tietze, for instance, commented: "At which point a human life or any life begins is a philosophical question, but I submit that throughout history the theologians and the jurists have always taken into account and have listened to the prevailing medical and biological consensus of the times, and I think this is still true. If a medical consensus develops and is maintained that pregnancy, and therefore life, begins at implantation, eventually our brethren from the other faculties will listen."[8] Alan Guttmacher, then president of the Planned Parenthood Federation, agreed, citing a British church that approved of anti-implantation contraceptive methods. He announced optimistically, "Obviously there are eminent theologians on our side even if it is proved that fertilization is not prevented by the [IUD]."[9]

The following year, the American Congress of Obstetricians and Gynecologists (ACOG) defined *conception* as the implantation of a fertilized ovum.[10] Under this medical definition, abortion cannot occur until the fertilized egg is implanted. Today the Life Issues Institute charges ACOG of conspiring to gain acceptability of contraceptive methods. Its Web site proclaims that under the 1965 medical definition of *conception,* doctors are deceitfully providing abortion using birth control methods. Willke writes: "Today a physician can truthfully call the IUD a 'contraceptive,' and mean that it prevents implantation in the wall of the uterus, while his patient, hearing him use the word, 'contraception,' will understand it to mean 'the prevention of the union of sperm and ovum.' And so, presto! An abortifacient is called a 'contraceptive,' and everybody is fooled. A classic example of double speak, or the perversion of language."[11]

Similar objections from antiabortion organizations that define the beginning of life as the moment of fertilization are common today.[12] But in 1965, the ACOG's redefinition of conception as the point of implantation was enough to give a green light to the development and distribution of the IUD as a method of contraception. Since the device was believed to work prior to implantation, it would not cause an abortion by this medical definition.

Although developers were relieved of the burden of having to address the abortion issue in their research and development, they were still sensitive to objections that women or doctors might raise to a method that would interfere with the implantation of a fertilized egg. Hugh Davis, inventor of the Dalkon Shield and a strong population control proponent, suggested in his 1971 book that physicians give the following response to clients who inquire about how the device works: "The IUD prevents pregnancy by preventing conception. The device inside the womb arouses natural body defenses, which cause the eggs and seed to dissolve and pass away as they do normally before the period comes."[13] Davis avoids using the specific terms *fertilization* and *implantation*, thus evading clarification of the exact point of the reproductive process at which the IUD intervenes. Providing ambiguous explanations to clients may have been a means of skirting the abortion question in a clinical setting during the 1960s and 1970s.

Gradually research on the IUD mechanism of action yielded new ideas about how the device prevents pregnancy. Studies showed that the foreign body in the uterus induced an immune response by the white blood cells, which destroyed the sperm and the fertilized ovum.[14] By the end of the 1970s, IUD researchers no longer considered the original idea that the IUD created a uterine environment inhospitable to implantation the most significant or plausible mechanism of action. Rather, they had come to view it as a possible secondary function to spermicidal and ovumcidal action.

During the late 1970s and early 1980s, the scientific community appears to have paid little attention to the device's contraceptive mechanism.[15] IUD developers' attention was presumably diverted from pursuing the precise physiological response because of other pressing items on the research agenda, such as testing copper-bearing devices and studying health risks associated with IUDs. More significant, there was little political pressure before the mid-1980s to specify whether IUDs prevent fertilization.

The Political Tide Turns against Family Planning Advocates
The rise of conservatism and the attendant opposition to family planning programs in the 1980s created a renewed interest in, and a need for, more

studies on the IUD's mechanism of action. A conservative constituency that had attempted unsuccessfully to reverse the 1973 legalization of abortion in the United States turned its attention to the global South as a new frontier to pursue its anti–reproductive rights agenda. Their efforts resulted in the gradual reduction of American involvement in promoting family planning abroad, starting with President Carter's replacement of U.S. Agency for International Development (USAID) executives with conservative Catholics, who subsequently dissolved USAID's Office of Population. This resulted in a significant decline in American foreign aid for contraceptive distribution. Religious groups and the political Right continued to build their power base to pursue culturally conservative policymaking in the United States that extended beyond the abortion issue. By the 1980s, the political New Right started using the "pro-life" banner to promote a complete set of conservative principles, central to which was the restoration of the traditional patriarchal family system and a sexual morality that forbid extramarital sex.[16]

The mid-1980s marked a time when international family planning supporters felt the American political tide turn dramatically against family planning services in the global South. The New Right's culminating success during this era was the 1984 institution of the Mexico City Policy, also known as the global gag rule. President Reagan's delegation to the U.N. Conference on Population in Mexico City announced that the United States would no longer provide funds to any agency that provided abortion services, counseling, or referrals. It thereby forbid organizations to offer information to clients on abortion or risk losing funding and hampering their birth control services as well. This new policy reversed the pro–family planning position the United States had followed for the past decade and a half. Early U.S. policies that had been driven by population control ideology were not without problems, but withholding funding to family planning programs at this time came as a serious setback to nongovernmental organizations and foreign governments that relied on U.S. aid to improve much-needed birth control services in the global South.[17]

In his 2003 memoir, *Under the Banyan Tree: A Population Scientists' Odyssey*, Sheldon Segal, recipient of the U.N. Population Award and a veteran of the Population Council and the Rockefeller Foundation, recounts an episode that happened just after James Buckley, head of the U.S. delegation to the Mexico City conference, announced the global gag rule.[18] As the audience left the meeting room, an American television anchorman started to interview the president of the Planned Parenthood Federation of America, Faye Wattleton, who expressed her dismay in the new policy that, she said, did not represent the American view at large. As Segal watched, John Willke, the religious leader quoted at the opening of this chapter, elbowed his way to the front of the crowd and into the camera's view.[19] When the anchorman asked him if he was satisfied with the U.S. position paper, Willke answered, "It was a good first step." In reply to the reporter's follow-up question on what the "next step" would be, Willke answered, "Now the United States has to stop all those abortions caused by contraceptives, like the pill and the IUD."[20]

Segal recounts his subsequent exchange with the same anchorman as follows: "When I was asked to comment, I did not hesitate to say that [Willke's] statement astonished me, not only because of its lack of scientific credibility, but because it revealed the true extent of his opposition to women's reproductive rights. It did not stop at abortion. It included contraception as well."[21] Here Segal refers to a strategy still commonly used by social conservatives: piggybacking their hostility to contraception on the antiabortion rhetoric. The following year, Segal and his colleagues published the first of a series of scientific reports that concluded that IUDs do not work by aborting embryos.[22] Whether his encounter with Willke directly motivated Segal to revitalize the study on the IUD's mechanism of action, I can only speculate. But as someone who dedicated his career to contraceptive development and distribution, he must have felt compelled to respond to antiabortionists' attack on the IUD.[23] The true mechanism of IUD's action was not the only thing at stake, however; the future of family planning policies and programs was as well.

Stabilizing the Antifertilization Theory: The Late 1980s

Following the Mexico City conference, the time was ripe for renewed studies of how IUDs work. Scientific developments, such as a recently discovered technique that detects small amounts of pregnancy-related hormone in urine samples, made it reasonable for researchers to reinvestigate the controversial physiological changes induced by the IUD.[24] Studies of the Norplant's mechanism of action had been done during the preceding few years, which may have also motivated similar studies on the IUD.[25] More important, strengthening scientific research that would refute the

construction of the IUD as an abortifacient and justifying it as a contraceptive method had suddenly become imperative for IUD supporters in the
political climate of the mid-1980s.

Supporters of the IUD understood that accusations that the device was an
abortifacient were based on the original hypothesis that the device worked
at the uterine level, that is, prohibiting a developing embryo from implant-
ing on the uterine wall. Scientists who had kept up with IUD research knew
that the anti-implantation mechanism was probably not the only mode of
action because studies conducted during the 1970s had suggested that this
foreign object in the uterus also induced physiological reactions that created a uterine environment inhospitable for sperm and ovum to survive.
It seemed to them that new scientific studies showing more definitively
that the device does not exert its antifertility effect by interfering with the
implantation of a fertilized egg were needed to overturn the old image.
Researchers who embarked on the mission to rescue the IUD from what
they believed was a misperception interpreted their task to be establishing
scientifically that no evidence of embryonic development could be found
in IUD users. They also sought to defend the antifertilization hypothesis by
gathering data that would strengthen the likelihood that the IUD stopped
pregnancy before the sperm could join the egg. Based on these premises,
a number of Population Council–affiliated scientists looked for signs of
developing embryos (or the lack thereof) in IUD users using three different
approaches.

The first set of studies aimed at discrediting the anti-implantation theory was initiated by Sheldon Segal, who searched for human chorionic gonadotropin (hCG), a hormonal substance produced by embryos around
the time of implantation—about seven days after fertilization. His 1985
study used a method resembling highly sensitive pregnancy tests, which
were conducted through daily blood and urine samples from IUD users
and control groups for at least one menstrual cycle. No hCG was detected
in Segal's thirty IUD users during the fertile period, suggesting there were
no developing embryos.[26] A third-party follow-up study in 1987 confirmed
that postovulatory hCG surges in IUD users were rare; it was observed in
only 1 among 107 menstrual cycles. Its authors concluded that the IUD
rarely acted as an anti-implantation method.[27] The argument in these studies is carefully crafted. Researchers were well aware that the hCG detection
method could tell only whether a fertilized egg could mature enough to

produce a detectable amount of hCG; it could not tell whether a sperm ever fertilized the egg. The studies claimed to disprove that IUDs abort a developing embryo in the uterus, and they did exactly that.

The second approach to supporting the antifertilization theory was to look for indications that sperm were severely incapacitated with an IUD in utero. Although this approach did not look for the existence of embryos, it accounted for the unlikelihood of a normal fertilization and development. In 1987, two Chilean scientists with close ties to the Population Council published a review of studies of sperm in IUD users that were conducted during the 1970s and early 1980s. Some studies had observed that spermatozoa are phagocytized, or engulfed by white blood cells, in the uterine cavity of IUD users. Others had found many sperm with their heads and tails separated.[28] Irvin Sivin of the Population Council reinforced these findings in a 1989 article by explaining that the toxic or spermicidal effect of copper likely caused sperm performance to deteriorate.[29] As with the hCG studies, these studies do not tell conclusively whether fertilization takes place; whether spermatozoa reach the fertilization site in sufficient numbers or retain their fertilizing capacity technically remains unknown. Nevertheless, observations of large numbers of debilitated sperm do suggest that they are less likely to reach the normal site of fertilization in the same number or condition as they do in non-IUD users, and thus that the device most likely inhibits fertilization.

The third approach to disproving the anti-implantation theory was to visually observe eggs under the microscope to look for signs of development.[30] Frank Alvarez of the Dominican Republic, who had collaborated with Segal on the hCG detection study, searched for eggs in the contents of the uterus and fallopian tubes of women who underwent sterilization surgery. Half of the eggs among the twenty-one recovered from noncontraceptive users who had had intercourse during the fertile period had been fertilized and showed normal embryonic development. Nine out of the fourteen eggs recovered from IUD users showed no development, suggesting that these eggs were not fertilized. The remaining five eggs from IUD users were categorized as showing abnormal or uncertain development. The authors could not say exactly whether these eggs had undergone fragmentation after being fertilized or had degenerated unfertilized.[31] The study also showed that the recovery rate of eggs (fertilized or not) from copper IUD users (30 percent) was substantially lower than the controls

(56 percent). These results suggested that IUDs generated uterine and fallopian tube environments that interfered with both successful fertilization and normal egg development and survival.

Since there was no reasonable means to prove that fertilization never occurs, supporters reasoned that IUDs are not abortifacient by presenting data that pointed to the unlikelihood of fertilization. Conclusions drawn from these studies managed to persuade the mainstream scientific community that the primary mechanism by which the IUD prevents pregnancy is by creating environmental changes in both the uterus and fallopian tubes that affect the fertilization process by inhibiting sperm and ova migration and survival. A sensible scientific consensus was built around this theory, and mainstream medical information outlets started to adopt this perspective. It would seem that those who supported the IUD as a legitimate contraceptive method had successfully negotiated the acceptability of the device among their colleagues.

The anti-implantation image, however, remained dominant in the public; thus, even people who were pro-choice continued to subscribe to it. As an example, in the 1988 *Webster* v. *Reproductive Health Services* ruling, Justice John Paul Stevens argued his case against an antiabortion Missouri provision stating that it unconstitutionally burdened users of IUDs and morning-after pills. He asserted that since Missouri "defines fetal life as beginning upon the fertilization of the ovum of a female by a sperm of a male," restrictive measures of abortion by implication would be applied to these particular contraceptive methods that "may operate to prevent pregnancy only after conception as defined in the statute,"[32] thereby unconstitutionally interfering with contraceptive choices. While clearly opposing an antichoice legislation, Justice Stevens inadvertently linked the IUD to abortion in a public statement. Shortly after, as if to put an end to what he viewed as mischaracterization of this contraceptive method, Irvin Sivin published an article, "IUDs Are Contraceptives, Not Abortifacients," in *Studies in Family Planning* in which he called the anti-implantation hypothesis of the device a "social myth."[33]

The Battle over the Womb

Mischaracterization of IUDs as an anti-implantation method is still common, more often than not made intentionally rather than as an inadvertent error. Not surprisingly, antiabortion leaders have blatantly ignored the antifertilization theory. But physicians who sympathize with their world-view and have joined them take a different approach; they challenge the idea through the medical discourse. As discussed in chapter 2, IUD develop-ers once perceived the womb as the battleground in the war against popula-tion during the 1960s. In the 1970s, the womb turned into a battlefield in the war against abortion. Since the 1980s, the uterus has been the point of contention between antichoice physicians, who aim to keep it device free, and IUD developers, who support the device's occupation of the womb. The reproductive organ has become a site of struggle where religious lead-ers and physicians wrestle to lay their claims on the knowledge of what actually happens inside it with an IUD in place.

Religious Leaders: Guards of the Womb

When the number of abortions in the United States rose after their legaliza-tion in 1973, some religious conservatives became increasingly convinced that contraception was to blame for the increase.[34] Cultural conservatives also accused a "contraceptive mentality" for promoting teenage promiscu-ity and sexual immorality.[35] As Rosalind Petchesky points out, the anti-abortion movement, rooted in conservative religious and cultural values, encompassed a desire to contain sexual activity to "patriarchally legitimate forms, those that reinforce heterosexual marriage and motherhood."[36] Thus, antiabortionists regard contraceptive use in general as the culprit for all aspects of what it views as sexual misconduct in its quest to preserve the traditional nuclear family. Curtailing sex education, suppressing teen-age sexuality and autonomy, and restricting the reproductive freedom of all women are items they have pursued on their agenda. By characterizing contraceptives as abortifacients and incorporating them in its opposition to abortion, the antiabortion movement discourages contraceptive use and helps perpetuate patriarchal control over women's bodies and lives.

The antiabortion movement also turned the womb into a locus of struggle that sometimes involved bizarre notions. The legalization of abor-tion coincided with the final phase of the losing war in Vietnam. Carol Mason argues, the psychological trauma and the demasculinization ef-fect of the lost war in Vietnam turned some Americans to the womb as a new battlefield. "Stopping baby killers" became the new crusade for them in order to stave off God's wrath so he would not strike at the new millennium.[37] The notion of abortion as a sin that must be stopped to achieve the Apocalypse generated antiabortion movements that increasingly resorted to violence. Besides the extreme notion of war against abortion, the strong religious framing of the antiabortion movement provided the New Right with an opportunity to justify its cause through moral absolutism. The group demonized communists, feminists, homosexuals, and liberal welfare advocates, while it idolized family, children, God, and what it viewed as "the American way." As Petchesky contends, abortion came to represent "all the satanic evils the right seeks . . . to destroy," while the fetus symbolized "the pristine and the innocent which must be protected and saved."[38] The uterus thus became the battlefield not only for a war against abortion, but also against liberal social movements. Within this context, a uterus containing an IUD signified not only baby killing, but also an invasion into political territory that the New Right was determined to guard from its opponents.

John Willke's testimony on the Life Issues Institute Web site conveys his determination to keep the uterus free of IUDs. In addition to misinforming his readers that 95 percent of scientific studies support the theory that the device works after fertilization, he intimidates women who might be considering IUD use by exaggerating the risk of infection and infertility. He describes in detail how uterine infections travel to the fallopian tubes, which "become badly damaged" and "scar shut," leaving the woman "sterile for life." He then affirms that IUDs are common health hazards. "I tell you," he writes, "I've seen it again and again through my years of being a physician. When we go against nature, sooner or later we pay the price."[39] Certainly risks associated with IUD use should not be ignored, but Willke completely dismisses the possibility of using the device safely. Determinedly, he continues: "How did these infections occur? Well, the womb was made to have only one object inside of it. That object is called a baby. . . . The IUD is a foreign body that just doesn't belong there . . . and that's what produces the problem."[40] Willke's attempt to keep Christian women from using an IUD amounts to a threat that if women "go against nature" (or "God"), they will suffer the consequences. By claiming expertise as a physician who "knows" and a religious leader who "cares," he seizes control over women's actions and wombs, safeguarding the organ/battlefield against foreign object invasion.

Willke does not hesitate to use violent metaphors to convince women not to use an IUD. He explains that the presence of an IUD damages the uterine lining and prevents implantation, but then he adds: "They may also work by poisoning the tiny human with the macrophage screen, or sterile pus that its presence produces." He underscores the distinct ways in which copper IUDs "kill": "Apparently some of the copper leaches or rusts off at a fairly steady rate inside of the womb and this may act as a low-grade poison, which helps to kill the tiny new human."[41] Willke appeals to female readers' moral consciousness by referring to the blastocyst (a newly fertilized egg) as the "tiny new human" and graphically portraying its "death." He has thus turned the IUD's mechanism of action into warfare and a killing field in the antiabortion discourse while at the same time he guards the womb by rhetorically eliminating any possibility that a Christian woman would "allow [an IUD] to be inserted."

Antiabortion Physicians on the Offense

What religious leaders like John Willke achieve by instilling guilt and fear, physicians who align with his worldview accomplish by publishing medical journal articles opposing the antifertilization theory of the IUD's mechanism of action. Joseph Spinnato's 1997 article in the *American Journal of Obstetrics and Gynecology* is an example of an attempt to rationalize opposition to IUD insertions in religious women.[42] He asserts that "substantial evidence exists supporting inhibition of implantation as a significant mechanism of action of the IUD."[43] In arguing that "there is not satisfactory evidence to conclude that a spermicidal prevention of fertilization is the exclusive method of action of IUDs," Spinnato undermines, reinterprets, or otherwise ignores existing studies that suggest that an IUD's primary mode of action precedes fertilization.[44] In addition, he expresses his discontent toward recent reviews and gynecological texts that refute, minimize, or do not mention interference with implantation when discussing the IUD's mechanisms of action. Spinnato then inflates the probability that the contraceptive method works after fertilization without referencing mainstream scientific reviews that suggest otherwise.

Sheldon Segal promptly stepped up to rebut Spinnato's claims. In his letter to the editor of the journal, Segal points out that Spinnato made selective references to past studies and ignored key articles that constitute the mainstream scientific consensus on how the contraceptive device prevents pregnancy. Criticizing Spinnato, Segal concludes: "It cannot escape a reader's attention that the Spinnato article brings the IUD into the abortion debate in the United States. Without introducing new data, it concludes that contraceptive IUDs act after fertilization, implying that they could be classified as abortifacients, although there is no factual basis for this categorization."[45]

Despite Segal's confutation, Spinnato managed to create an impression that there was a scientific disagreement over the issue and to provide a published reference to cite for other like-minded physicians. Some have followed suit and carried on the dispute within the medical community. Walter Larimore, for instance, criticizes Timothy Canavan, who advised physicians to inform patients that the IUD prevents conception and is not an abortifacient in a 1999 article, "Appropriate Use of the Intrauterine Device," in *American Family Physician*.[46] Citing Spinnato's article, Larimore remarked in his letter to the editor that there was not enough evidence that fertilization was completely omitted and that therefore it would be violating the female patient's autonomy if this information were withheld. In response, Canavan dissented, maintaining that the risk of postfertilization action is so remote that it is not worthwhile mentioning it to patients, just as making reference to the remote chance of death when performing a routine surgical procedure is overkill.[47] The editors of *American Family Physician* decided that because the issue was so emotionally charged, the electronic version of the patient education handout on the IUD needed to be modified to acknowledge the controversy. It now alludes to the possibility that an IUD may cause the thinning of the lining of the uterine wall, an expression that has become a euphemism for preventing implantation.[48]

Preemptive Arguments against Natural Embryonic Losses

The debate around the IUD's mechanism of action may be gradually shifting toward whether or not the device is responsible for the loss of embryos beyond what would have been lost without the use of a contraceptive method. General studies of early pregnancy factor (EPF) detection suggest that many fertilized eggs are lost before they reach the implantation stage, that is, within about a week of ovulation. Depending on the study, the ratio of preimplantation embryonic loss in noncontracepters ranges from 17 to 36 percent.[49] Some researchers cite a figure as high as 30 to 70 percent to describe the number of embryos that are "lost before or at the time of implantation, without women being aware that they were pregnant."[50] In addition, a study of early loss after implantation shows that 25 percent of fertilized eggs that appeared to have implanted were lost before the sixth week of pregnancy.[51]

These studies point out that women regularly pass fertilized eggs or miscarry (or "abort" if we follow the definition of abortion put forth by antiabortionists) without their knowledge. IUD supporters, then, could conceivably make an argument that the chances of losing an embryo are much lower in IUD users as compared to nonusers since the device makes fertilization much more difficult. Reminding women that their normal reproductive function involves natural embryonic losses can also offer an explanation of their physiological processes that would not hold them guilty of causing an abortion with a contraceptive method. Yet IUD advocates have not done so, possibly fearing that admitting that fertilization can happen in rare cases would undermine their position. The only meek attempt I have seen is made by Irvin Sivin in his 1989 article, which notes, "No studies show that IUDs destroy developing embryos at rates higher than those found in women who are not using contraceptives."[52]

In fact, it appears that it is the antichoice physicians who anticipated such reasoning and preempted it by arguing the contrary. Joseph Stanford and Rafael Mikolajczyk's 2002 study claims to have calculated the proportion of embryonic losses for which IUDs are uniquely accountable. They apply mathematical modeling to existing data and compute rates of estimated postfertilization embryonic loss that can be attributed to the effects of the device after natural spontaneous embryonic losses are accounted for.[53] In addition to the copper-releasing IUD, for which enough studies exist to suggest that the metal acts as a spermicide, the authors investigated hormone-releasing IUDs, whose mechanism is less understood and somewhat ambiguous. The data from previous studies that they analyzed were by no means complete. Yet they managed to present an estimated number of embryonic losses attributed to the hormone-releasing device: 0.2 to 1.0 per woman per year. The authors claim to have shown that even if the device works predominantly by preventing fertilization, "a very potent postfertilization effect is required to achieve the observed low rates of clinical pregnancy."[54]

Stanford and Mikolajczyk present their study as being motivated by patients' interests: "[We] believe that these results have important implications for the counseling of women and couples who are considering the use of the IUD."[55] Yet another important role that their article plays is the

canny characterization of IUDs as responsible for "induced" loss of fertilized eggs. Publishing such a study in the *American Journal of Obstetrics and
Gynecology* clearly has the effect of destabilizing the image of the IUD as a
predominantly antifertilization method, an image the device's advocates
have worked hard to cultivate, as well as forestalling the argument the pro-
choice side could have made that without an IUD in place women regularly
pass fertilized eggs. It appears that IUD opponents have tightened their grip
around the uterine battleground.

The Biopolitical Script of the Religious Woman

Anti-IUD physicians' efforts to reproach a well-accepted contraceptive
technology on the basis that it might induce abortion has been accompanied by a representation of an implicated user who is deeply worried
about knowingly terminating life. To justify their concerns about the device's mechanism of action and the doctor-patient interactions around it,
scientists who argue on behalf of the postfertilization IUD action theory
have enlisted women who have moral objections against such a device. In
effect, the discourse of an abortifacient device has been co-configured with
an ideal of the religious woman, as well as distinct ways to govern her body.

The Co-Configuration of an Abortifacient and Women with Moral Objections
Authors of articles that support the anti-implantation hypothesis profess
to have an altruistic motive for publishing their opinions: women, and
religious women in particular, would want to know if the device aborts,
and their choice will be at stake if they do not have a full scientific understanding of the IUD's mechanism of action. In fact, the viewpoint that
early embryonic loss cannot be ruled out would not have much importance without women who care about such issues. Not surprisingly, scientific papers by antiabortion advocates foreground women who morally
object to a postfertilization method. Spinnato, for instance, begins his
article by stating, "For many patients, decision-making regarding contraception is influenced by beginnings-of-life moral and religious considerations."[56] Larimore also contends that "[possible postfertilization action]
would be especially important for patients with moral objections." He follows this up with a warning to women's physicians: "If the potential effect violates the moral requirements of a woman and she is not informed

of the possibility, then this failure to disclosure seriously jeopardizes her autonomy."[57]

I am not critiquing the notion that some women would prefer not to use a contraceptive method that works primarily by preventing implantation. What I want to emphasize is that the representation of the conservative religious woman is what grants value to scientific papers that assert that an IUD user might destroy an embryo. The conservative religious woman, who is likely to reject methods that may permit fertilization, is a discursive figure coproduced with the notion that the IUD is abortifacient. She is mobilized within the anti-IUD discourse as a spokesperson for physicians' antagonism against what they refer to as postfertilization contraceptive methods and an authenticator of objections to presenting the device to patients as an antifertilization contraceptive method.

Reconfiguring Women's Experiences of Pregnancy
The dispute over the IUD's mechanism of action has consistently ignored the fact that women usually do not detect the moment of fertilization or implantation and thus often do not experience themselves as being pregnant at this stage. Historically, women's subjective knowledge about their bodies played a much more significant role in the ontology of pregnancy than did medical accounts of reproductive physiology.[58] A journal kept by a nineteenth-century middle-class American woman, for instance, shows that some women relied on tracking their periods and their own intuitions about their physical state as a means to establish pregnancy.[59] Mary Pierce Poor's diary shows that she fretted about possibly being pregnant when she felt ill or her menstruation was late. Following some of these occasions, she wrote with relief in her diary or in a letter to her husband that her suspicions were proven wrong (for she had menstruated or possibly had an early miscarriage). On other occasions, she was kept in suspense longer until there were other signs that convinced her she was indeed pregnant. The bottom line is that women used to obtain proof of pregnancy through their embodied experiences.

Over-the-counter pregnancy test kits now allow women to privately find out with more certainty whether they are pregnant before other obvious signs appear. Until a few years ago, however, the timing when women confirmed their pregnancies had not changed significantly since Victorian times. Until recently, pregnancy test manufacturers usually recommended that women take the test about a week or so after a missed period when the level of hCG in the urine was most likely elevated enough to be detectable. This coincided with the moment when a Victorian woman who kept track of her menstrual periods would have started to suspect that she might be pregnant. Thus, the impetus to test for pregnancy was linked to her knowledge of her own body. Although occasionally women attest to "feeling" pregnant during earlier weeks, their pregnancies were usually not confirmed until testing around six weeks into their pregnancies.

Owing to recent improvements in the sensitivity of the tests, kits now allow pregnancy testing five days before a missed period, around the time of implantation.[60] A woman who wants to find out whether she is pregnant as soon as possible can now purchase this knowledge over the counter before she experiences any bodily signs. Because women's stakes in pregnancy, whether wanted or unwanted, typically are high, it is understandable that some want an answer as soon as possible. Nevertheless, some individuals would likely feel disconnected from a positive test result that did not correspond to their physical sensations. Like these new pregnancy test kits, the debate over the hypothetical frequency of instances of fertilization and preimplantation loss in IUD users thoroughly displaces women's subjective experiences of the beginning of their pregnancy since it forces women to view themselves as pregnant before any signs have appeared.

A woman who wants to test for pregnancy as early as possible may welcome the technoscientifically mediated notion of the pregnant self. The conservative religious woman, who is expected to refuse a so-called abortifacient contraceptive, however, is *constrained* to a disembodied understanding of her pregnancy that starts at an undetectable moment of fertilization. Furthermore, she is obliged to adhere to the notion that her embryos were viable if it were not for the IUD. As I noted, without subjects who subscribe to these views, arguments that foreground women's objections to a contraceptive method that may in rare cases permit fertilization are useless. Intriguingly, Stanford and Mikolajczyk, who estimated the number of "induced" embryonic losses in IUD users, are coauthors of another study that claims that the majority of women do subscribe to this disembodied knowledge of pregnancy. Their survey, which was conducted in Spain, asked women whether it was important for them to distinguish natural embryonic losses from those caused by birth control.[61] The wording of the questionnaire, intentionally or not, was value laden: "natural" suggested "good" and "acceptable," whereas an effect of birth control implied "bad." Confronted by a survey that essentially asked them to make a moral judgment, 58.7 percent of all respondents stated that they distinguish the two. The same survey also reported that 40 percent of the women indicated that they would not use a method that works after fertilization.

As Theodore Porter argued, quantification "helps to produce knowledge independent of the particular people who make it," giving information an aura of objectivity.[62] I would add that through statistical representation, women who would refuse a contraceptive method are transformed into an ontological reality. Stanford and Mikolajczyk's study, which proclaims to have objectively measured the proportion of women who feel morally bound to avoid certain kinds of technologies, bolsters anti-IUD physicians' claim that since it matters to women, physicians need to inform their patients that the device might induce embryonic losses. Such information, however, compels women to conceptually distinguish natural reproductive processes from artificial destruction of an embryo, even though this distinction is neither observable nor subjectively experienced. This perspective on the body that deems "induced" embryonic loss to be a morally accountable material reality obliges women who ascribe to certain religious values to remove themselves from situations that involve remote possibility of an unintentional termination of a pregnancy. The "religious woman" then is simultaneously constructed through the scientific discourse and *governed at a distance* through the discursive articulation of her as the IUD refuser.[63]

Informed Consent as a Form of Governance

Antiabortion physicians also appropriated an existing form of governance to their end. Informed consent was built into IUD insertion practices as a response to the controversy over the method's health risks to women; informed consent provided a way to ensure that users conformed to safety standards. Anti-IUD physicians have altered the discourse of patients' rights and women's choice, which was originally advanced by feminists who advocated for informed consent, to govern the practices of fellow physicians and, through them, women's bodies.

Spinnato, for example, argues, "The prescription or marketing of IUDs that consciously understate or omit the likelihood of [anti-implantation] is deceptive and fails current standards of informed consent."[64] Since not

all physicians feel that it is necessary to inform their patients of the remote chance of a postfertilization effect, the author spends a considerable
amount of space trying to persuade fellow physicians to abide by the practice he hopes to see implemented. He writes:

On a physician-patient level these are more than mere issues of semantics; they are
ones of morality, personal choice, and informed consent. . . . If the mechanism of action of an IUD violates the moral requirements of the patient, failure to disclose this
information seriously jeopardizes her autonomy. . . . If information is deliberately
withheld or misstated regarding the action of IUDs, an unethical deception occurs.
Failure to disclose information that might lead a patient to choose a different mode
of treatment can be unethical. It would seem clear that failure to inform patients of
the likely postfertilization mechanism of action is a failure of informed consent.[65]

In addition, Spinnato holds that a woman who learns of the postfertilization action of the IUD may later experience a "psychologic conse-
quence," which includes "guilt, anger, depression, and a sense that she has
been violated by the provider."[66] His language comes close to threatening
physicians who ignore his plea and accusing them of sexual assault, which
the word *violate* suggests. Not accidentally, the symptoms the patient is
presumed to exhibit are also ones that rape victims often experience.

By inciting fear of patient complaints and preaching moral obligation,
antiabortion physicians recruit fellow doctors to assume the role of religious leaders while posing as medical experts. Once again the representation of a woman with a moral consciousness, who will be extremely upset
with even the slightest chance of an early embryonic loss, upholds the argument for a "full disclosure." Meanwhile, naturally occurring embryonic
losses are not mentioned, and women who may not care to be given immaterial information are not taken into account. When a doctor presents a
woman with a notion that a contraceptive method may pass fertilized eggs,
the patient is put in a position where she is asked to make a moral choice
rather than choose a contraceptive method. The anticipated outcome is
that some women will be persuaded to reconsider acquiring the device.

In this context, informed consent, or what antiabortion physicians per-
ceive as full disclosure, namely, one that includes the remote possibility
of fertilization, functions as a form of governance over women's bodies
against IUD insertion. Their repeated efforts to recruit health care practitioners to adopt the postfertilization version of informed consent reflect
the reality that doctors have significant power over women's contraceptive
decisions. Because physicians encounter many different women in their

practices, it can be anticipated that women from many walks of life will be caught off guard and made to feel judged by their health care providers. Thus, although IUD opponents emphasize concern for religious women's autonomy, the insertion protocol they advocate results in governing all women at a distance.

Misappropriating Choice

While anti-IUD physicians consistently emphasize religious women's autonomy in order to support their position on full disclosure, it is questionable how genuinely they speak for the best interest of every woman. An insensitive statement from one such physician reveals his scant commitment to women's welfare and his disregard for women of color in particular. In his article, Spinnato makes a statement reminiscent of the population controllers of the 1960s after he asserted that all health care providers, including those in the global South who may be religious, should be made aware of the postfertilization actions of IUDs: "These are issues of no minor consequences to global population control. IUDs are economical. Their insertion can be easily taught. Unlike barrier or oral contraceptives, *they require less motivation and virtually no patient compliance* [emphasis added]."[67]

As I discussed in chapter 2, developers initially praised the IUD as suitable for controlling population growth because it could be imposed on women who were unmotivated to contracept. Since then, however, IUD advocates have ceased using such patronizing expressions as they reshaped their discourse in response to feminist critique. In comparison, it is apparent that this antichoice physician, writing in 1997, was unaware or dismissive of feminist opposition against treating women of the global South as passive targets of population control. He appropriated the language of women's choice toward a particular end: to discourage IUD use by American women, while approving population control in the global South and showing no true regard for the feminist struggles to improve reproductive self-determination. On the contrary, IUD supporters gradually and successfully coalesced their position with feminists.

The IUD as Reproductive Choice

As IUD supporters adjusted their neo-Malthusian discourse to improve global acceptability of this contraceptive technology, they gradually adopted feminist approaches and language. And they did so much more skillfully than the inconsistent way in which antiabortion physicians appropriated "women's choice." The so-called war on choice also became one of the common points of agreement for feminists and IUD researchers as they joined efforts to promote birth control.

The Evolution of Alliances between Neo-Malthusians and Feminists

The alliance between feminists and neo-Malthusians in fact dates back to Margaret Sanger, who originally was a radical socialist feminist advocating birth control and sexual pleasure as women's rights. Around the mid-1910s, Sanger abandoned the explosive sexual component of her movement and recast birth control as a medical issue while she also turned to neo-Malthusians and eugenicists for support. As Carole McCann contends, Sanger was a pragmatic activist who garnered support for birth control by appealing to the interests of various social strata and whose movement evolved through "conflicted coalitions with other social groups within the shifting political terrain of the period."[68] During the pre–World War II period in particular, eugenicists' desire to restrict the reproduction of racial minorities coalesced with Sanger's goal to increase contraceptive access for the poor. While the United States was recovering from the Great Depression, Sangerists also argued that family planning was essential for the nation's economic recovery plan to be effective and that birth control services were essential for protecting women's health.[69]

McCann argues that when the dominant concept around fertility control moved to planned parenthood, child spacing, and family planning, it divorced birth control from feminist critiques of male dominance and masculinized the movement by allowing men to take over the administration of organizations such as Planned Parenthood. Dennis Hodgson and Susan Watkins present a slightly different perspective, noting that as the codirector of the International Planned Parenthood Federation (IPPF) from 1952 to 1959, Sanger "imprinted it with her feminist belief that birth control was essential for women's freedom."[70] At the very least, during the mid-twentieth century, Sanger and IPPF shared ideological and demographic goals: that birth control must be brought to the masses to reduce fertility and thereby benefit individual women and their smaller families, as well as alleviate social problems.

The neo-Malthusian movement after World War II was also strongly colored by eugenicist and imperialist prejudices against women of color and the global South. Prominent members of the neo-Malthusian establishment often endorsed coercive and semicoercive measures to accomplish population control.[71] With the advent of the second wave of the women's movement during the 1960s, feminist criticisms around coercive population control programs began to rise, particularly from the leftist or radical feminists. Women's health activists' suspicions toward neo-Malthusianism and the pharmaceutical industry spread as health risks associated with pill and IUD use became public during the late 1960s and 1970s. Liberal feminists were still in support of promoting birth control, but overall, the alliance between feminists and neo-Malthusians was attenuated during these two decades.

While feminists distrusted the neo-Malthusian movement, neo-Malthusians attempted to adopt a mildly feminist stance that advocated for women's well-being. As early as 1966, Population Council president Bernard Berelson stated that the "quality of service is of critical importance" and that patient education was not to be underestimated.[72] He made this assertion in response to women's unexpected resistance to IUD distribution projects in the global South. Hence, he was suggesting that women had to be won over, rather than coerced, in order to improve contraceptive dissemination. Sexism nevertheless still ran deep. Adrienne Germain, who worked at the Population Council and the Ford Foundation's population office in the early 1970s, was astonished at how men in the office talked about "users" and "accepters" "as though women weren't human."[73]

But as external criticisms against population control spread, neo-Malthusians carefully revised their language. For instance, John D. Rockefeller III wrote in the 1976 annual report of the Population Council: "We simply can no longer regard women in developing countries as statistics, merely as 'users' or 'acceptors,' but we must see them in all of their full and many-sided dimensions as human beings."[74] Feminists within the organization also worked toward changing the fundamentally neo-Malthusian activities to women-centered ones. For example, Judith Bruce, whose primary responsibility was to develop programs on the roles and status of women, instituted the quality-of-care framework that prioritizes client satisfaction. By 1990 the quality-of-care principle was formally adopted by the organization's overseas projects.[75] Bruce also emphasized the importance of the broader system of power within which women make reproductive choices as part of their survival strategies. She sought to revise contraceptive developers' narrow focus on women's perception of the technology, which did not take into account gender roles, cultural practices, and women's social statuses that directly or indirectly shaped the range of birth control practices that women could consider.[76]

Despite these improvements on the part of former population control advocates, according to Hodgson and Watkins, the division between neo-Malthusians and feminists widened during the 1980s. The global gag rule instituted in 1984 did not immediately bring them together either. Feminists who felt that Reagan's anti-Malthusian stance was a step forward for recasting reproduction as a health issue rather than a population and development issue welcomed the U.S. delegates' stance that "population was a neutral phenomenon" rather than a critical pathway toward modernization. The neo-Malthusians, who had always avoided abortion as an expensive and politically problematic method of birth control, did not react immediately to the antiabortion measure.

The alliance of feminists and neo-Malthusians was reassembled in earnest by the common ground established at the 1994 U.N. International Conference on Population and Development (ICPD) in Cairo. Since the 1980s, women's health activist groups such as the International Women's Health Coalition, Women's Global Network for Reproductive Rights, and Development Alternatives with Women had been working against both abusive population control programs and efforts to force women to bear unwanted children while engaging state policies, aid programs, and international organizations.[77] During the early 1990s, these feminist nongovernmental organizations started working toward the Cairo conference with the backing of Nafis Sadik, then head of the U.N. Population Fund (UNFPA), who advised them to work together with environmentalists and mainstream family planning groups. The coalition of women's health activists articulated new directions for population policies based on the goals of health, empowerment, and human rights instead of demographically motivated contraceptive distribution. For instance, in their 1994 book *Population Policies Reconsidered,* Gita Sen, Adrienne Germain, and Lincoln Chen declared that although population stabilization is a desirable goal, it does not warrant compulsion; that contraception is an individual human right, not for aggregate population control; and that women's empowerment is essential for achieving low fertility.[78]

Women's health activists' efforts were successful to the extent that the issues feminists brought up, such as human rights and reproductive rights, women's empowerment, reproductive and sexual health, and a woman-centered approach to fertility control became central concepts in the Program of Action documented in the Cairo meeting.[79] The Vatican's opposition to any references to abortion, however, weakened passages on reproductive and sexual rights. Its extremely conservative position also made the population constituency's support for birth control appear progressive, making them allies of the women's groups. The battle over abortion resulted in drawing the conference's attention away from women's groups' concerns that fundamental inequity and economic and political realities were the major source of infringement on reproductive rights.[80] As a result, the Cairo Consensus that was approved by a diverse group of ICPD participants, including population control constituencies, women's rights activists, and the Catholic church, fell short of pushing for fundamental changes to overthrow social inequities that hindered women's rights.

Although the Cairo Consensus endorsed a new framework for a woman-centered approach to population policy on the surface, it effectively settled on a middle ground, where the language could be appropriated for varying objectives.[81] For instance, "women's empowerment," which feminists advocated as vital for reproductive self-determination, was interpreted for policymaking purposes as an outcome of giving easier access to contraception. Organizations such as the Population Council and UNFPA supported the need for an overall improvement in health care and education for girls and women. But they also construed the woman-centered agenda somewhat narrowly for their contraceptive development and distribution programs, reasoning that increasing the variety of contraceptive offerings would better ensure that women's reproductive needs would be met.[82] At the very least, contraceptive developers positioned themselves as allies of women's health activists and as being part of the solution for achieving women's empowerment in the new discourse of woman-centered reproductive health.

Whether the Cairo Consensus was a victory for women is still debated and warrants an extended analysis. Some positive changes in programs in the global South have been reported, although the examples of success are by no means generalizable.[83] Matthew Connelly, a historian of demography, contends that the Cairo program marked the end of population control as a global movement, but some feminist scholars have been doubtful.[84] Health activist Betsy Hartmann, for instance, believed that neo-Malthusians colluded with environmental activists and exploited feminist language to continue pursuing demographically oriented endeavors.[85] Hodgson and Watkins, who traced the history of the alliances between feminists and neo-Malthusians, also suspected that the coalition would be rather fragile.[86] Saul Halfon, who studied how the Cairo Consensus was negotiated, observes that by building on the understanding that individual empowerment provides a solution to societal problems, the population discourse increasingly construes female subjects as individual consumers. He cautions that new rhetoric that equates women's empowerment with contraceptive market reform might be detrimental to a woman-centered approach to reproductive health in the global South.[87]

Neutralizing the IUD as Contraceptive Choice

The language of woman-centered family planning helped shift the discourse around contraceptive technologies from an instrument to achieve population control to a tool for women to fulfill their goals. The idea that women need to be able to choose from a range of fertility control methods, however, is not new. As early as the mid-1960s, the rhetoric around the IUD had already shifted away from casting it as the panacea for curbing population growth and instead favored it as an option in a "cafeteria" of offerings.[88] As Nelly Oudshoorn points out, when contraceptive developers conceded that an ideal contraceptive that fits all could not be developed, they readily took a new position, which claimed the need for a wide variety of contraceptive methods that would suit the world's diverse population and different living conditions and circumstances. This reform, she contends, helped contraceptives move into a postmodern phase, where differences among women offered opportunities for building new markets.[89]

Initially, however, giving women more contraceptive choices was conceptualized as a way to secure overall fertility reduction.[90] During the intervening years, as the discourse around international development gradually recognized the important social and economic roles women play, representations of female contraceptive users also changed from passive accepters of family planning who needed to be educated and persuaded to use birth control to that of voluntary family planning program clients whose broader needs must be respected. The post-Cairo population rhetoric further repositioned women as active agents who seek to control their fertility with a method that best suits their needs. In this context, the cafeteria offering has been reframed as serving women's unmet needs for reproductive health care.

The new paradigm effectively reconfigured the IUD as one of many contraceptive options women actively seek out, superseding the past rhetoric that hailed the device as the one-time intervention method that would help limit population growth. The device is now presented as a good choice for many women who use contraceptives, the availability of which would lead to their empowerment by enabling them to control their fertility.[91] The discursive rearrangement effectively neutralized the device: it is no longer a contra-feminist method that is used as a tool for imposing contraception on women, but rather a profeminist device that assists women in achieving their goals.

Former neo-Malthusian IUD developers are not the only ones who subscribe to this characterization. Gloria Feldt, former president of the Planned Parenthood Federation of America and a self-proclaimed feminist, recounts meeting "Maria," a Mexican mother of five small children whose husband objected to her taking the pill despite her apparent physical weakness. When her friends suggested an IUD to control her fertility without her husband's knowledge, Maria visibly brightened. "I knew," Feldt writes, "I was witnessing a quiet revolution."[92] Feldt's position reinforces contraceptive researchers' stance that having access to a variety of birth control technologies opens up the path to empowerment for women.[93]

Allies during the War on Choice

Feldt's support for the global availability of contraceptives is strongly tied to pro-choice feminism. Pro-choice feminists have fought against American right-wing extremists' all-inclusive opposition (from abortion to contraception) to reproductive rights. Not all feminists are in agreement with their approach, however. Mainstream pro-choice feminists' uncritical embrace of all contraceptives and narrow focus on protecting legal rights and practical access to abortion are questioned by feminists of color who unite around the concept of reproductive justice. These feminists criticize the pro-choice paradigm for failing to address the deprivation of reproductive choice that underprivileged women of color experience.[94] They are skeptical of pro-choice organizations such as Planned Parenthood, viewing them as extensions of the population control movement that favors legislation that may be detrimental to women of color.

Andrea Smith calls for a reproductive justice movement that would be "truly liberatory for all women," that is, independent of the single-issue-driven pro-choice framework.[95] Among the concerns she raises against pro-choice groups are that they tend to advocate all contraceptives as choice while failing to maintain "a critical perspective on dangerous or potentially dangerous contraceptives" and that informed consent has not been rigorously practiced in the application of these methods that are often problematically promoted in communities of color.[96] Smith specifically refers to Norplant and Depo-Provera as potentially dangerous and abusive methods. Given her concern toward long-acting provider-controlled methods that are difficult to discontinue at the user's will, it would not be far-fetched to extrapolate that the IUD would fall within the same category of potentially harmful methods that she says are uncritically supported by pro-choice feminists and disproportionately offered to underprivileged women.

Notwithstanding, the war on choice has drawn IUD researchers and pro-choice feminists closer. In his memoir, Sheldon Segal endorses the Cairo Consensus and advocates for better health care and education for girls and women and improving the social status of female citizens. Predictably he backs contraceptive development for women's empowerment while arguing that more effective methods will "advance reproductive freedom and reduce the number of abortions performed in the United States and around the world."[97] Expressing his frustrations toward the global gag rule, the Vatican, and George W. Bush's administration's avoidance of population issues at U.N. conferences, he urges diverse parties to unite against anticontraceptive movements. He writes: "The zealots who would deny women their reproductive freedom should be opposed by a unified coalition of concerned scientists, feminist leaders, policy advocates, and others working together for sexual equality and women's health and empowerment and for clearer understanding of the global consequences of population growth."[98] Segal's statement represents a strong belief in the reduction of overall global fertility, while he also adopts pro-choice feminist goals and discourses. He is not hesitant to align himself with feminists and call himself an advocate of gender equality. In the context of the U.S. and international war on choice, IUD developers appropriately claim themselves to be allies of feminists.

In today's political climate, it is conceivable that if antiabortionists successfully promote widely the notion that IUDs and other methods are abortifacient this could create an obstacle for donors, governments, and health care providers who offer contraceptives to their clients. The current Planned Parenthood president, Cecile Richards, has campaigned to overturn the rule issued by the U.S. Department of Health and Human Services during the last months of George W. Bush's administration that allows any member of a health care institution's workforce to refuse to provide health care services based on his or her personal beliefs, without ensuring that patients' needs will in some way be met. Reproductive health advocates are particularly wary of such a law that allows doctors and pharmacists to refrain from giving patients information about contraceptives or dispensing them.

Such legislation would most likely have the greatest impact on Plan B, the postcoital emergency contraceptive, which is in the middle of a similar, and far more visible, struggle over its precise mechanism of action as the IUD.[99] But access to all contraceptive methods would become precarious since a personal objection suffices to withhold information, a prescription, or the medication itself. In light of persistent antichoice movements in the United States, the former neo-Malthusian contraceptive developers' efforts to build scientific consensus around the antifertilization theory of the mechanism of contraceptive technologies could assist pro-choice feminist activism by undermining post-fertilization hypotheses that motivate anti-abortion physicians and pharmacists to refuse to provide contraception.

The Biopolitics of the IUD's Mechanism of Action

Although antiabortion physicians hold that they are specifically concerned about religious women, the implications of their claims reach far beyond this group. Their deliberate assertion that the IUD is an abortifacient has the potential of altering how physicians inform their patients about contraceptive options; it may influence accessibility to contraceptives for all women; it may change the ways women make choices about birth control; and it could have an impact on domestic and international policies surrounding reproductive health care. Representations of contraceptive mechanisms of action thus have biopolitical implications that reach nationwide and beyond.

Because science has cultural authority over "the truth," it is mobilized in a number of debates that are political in nature. Even John Willke, who openly appeals to fear and guilt in his effort to dissuade women from using an IUD, invokes science to legitimize his position. Antichoice physicians who publish in peer-reviewed journals use scientific arguments to try to weaken the claim that IUDs are a contraceptive, not an abortifacient. The device's supporters have always regarded science as the arbiter of problems that have underlying ideological issues. In the 1960s, they put their faith in the medical definition of conception to detract opposition. More recently they have made efforts to produce definitive studies that support the IUD's antifertilization hypothesis and tried to use scientific arguments to settle the abortion question.

Yet relying on science as an arbitrator of a political conflict has run into problems of late. Bruno Latour points out that even when there is a strong consensus among scientists on a particular issue, a few scientists can open up a scientific controversy by contradicting the conclusion.[100] An "artificially maintained scientific controversy" can give the impression to the public that experts on the issue at hand disagree. Recently mainstream scientific views that involve significant political stakes, such as the human impact on global warming and health effects of environmental toxins, have been challenged by a few scientists who argue that these correlations have not been scientifically confirmed. Scientific dissent has become a common technique that those who oppose regulations turn to. In the case of global warming, minority scientific opinions have been used to deny the seriousness of environmental problems and weaken policymaking efforts toward regulating greenhouse gas emissions. Similar interventions have also been made against regulations that limit the use of synthetic chemicals.[101]

The case of the IUD is comparable to Latour's notion of manufactured controversy. Expert researchers familiar with the IUD built a scientific consensus that it works predominantly by preventing fertilization, only to be challenged by a few dissenting scientists who contradicted the dominant view by reappropriating the data and turned the consensus into an unsettled matter. As is the case with climate change and environmental health, the dispute over how to represent the device's function is not a debate in and of itself; it is an ideological conflict veiled by science.

The disagreement over the IUD's mechanism of action is not easily resolvable scientifically or ideologically. Arguably most scientists would conclude that the device impairs sperm mobility, making fertilization unlikely and halting pregnancy sometime before the embryo is formed or descends into the uterus. They would most likely agree that fertilization, if it takes place at all, is very rare. To find out precisely how rare is difficult: it would require additional funds, researchers, and facilities; improved technology that detects fertilization precisely and efficiently; and experimental subjects, namely women, who would submit themselves to strict experimental protocols and invasive procedures. Hundreds of women, many of them from the global South, have already surrendered their bodies to invasive scrutiny during the 1980s for research on the IUD's mechanism of action: seventy-five women from the Dominican Republic provided daily blood samples for one menstrual cycle;[102] forty American women collected daily first-morning urine samples for three months;[103] and 171 women from the Dominican Republic and Chile had daily urine sample testing and cervical exams before receiving surgical sterilization and having the contents of their removed reproductive organs flushed in search of signs of fertilized eggs.[104] It would be antithetical to the feminist cause to ask more women to participate in invasive studies, even if more refined data could strengthen a pro-choice argument.[105]

Besides, the critical argument is over how the IUD should be represented, not just exactly how it works. The conflict is irreconcilable because one party uses the medical classification of conception that defines implantation as the start of pregnancy in calling the method a contraceptive, while the other party insists on the definition of fertilization as the beginning of life in identifying the device an abortifacient. Hence, as long as anti-abortionists are adamant that a contraceptive method is an abortifacient if fertilization ever occurs, IUD supporters will find little recourse in using science as the arbitrator.

Continuing the debate might not seem beneficial to the pro-choice side since opponents could take advantage of it to promote the idea that IUDs somehow cause abortions, even though fertilization is arguably rare in IUD users. In spite of that, IUD supporters have no choice but to try to maintain control over the definition of the device's mechanism of action. The struggle is not merely about whose representation is more accurate, but who will seize power over the body. Characterizing the device as a postfertilization method renders technological intervention in the body morally impermissible, whereas an understanding that the device predominantly prohibits the joining of the sperm and the egg precludes it from the moral conundrum of abortion. The mechanism of action of any contraceptive method is indeed a case in which scientific claims exercise biopower.

While the stake in the battle over knowledge is high, pro-choice feminists cannot rely solely on science to be the arbitrator for their quest to secure contraceptives as acceptable technologies. Reproductive rights are always going to be a political struggle that must be fought on many fronts, including scientific representation of contraceptive methods, law and policymaking, and cultural changes. Feminists and IUD supporters can align themselves in advocating policies that facilitate contraceptive accessibility domestically and overseas.

While the device's historical roots as an imposable fertility control method should be remembered to circumvent abusive practices, collaboration between feminists and IUD supporters has led to the conversion of the IUD discourse from population control to women's contraceptive choice. The scientific debate around the IUD's mechanism of action is an important ingredient in this discursive transformation. Meanwhile, IUD opponents' active challenges have elevated the visibility of their biopolitical script and embedded the language of the "abortifacient device" into the material-discursive construct of this contraceptive technology. The "religious woman/IUD refuser" has become just as much a part of the multiple scenarios embodied by this heterogeneous technology as have the "masses," the "moms," and the women who are "empowered" by birth control options.

5 "Keep Life Simple": Body/Technology Relationships in Racialized Global Contexts

After the birth of my second child in 2005, I had my second IUD inserted. This time it was a Mirena, which releases a synthetic progestin, levonorgestrel, from an intrauterine capsule and prevents pregnancy for five years without replacement. The device is one of the most effective contraceptive methods, comparable to surgical sterilization. In clinical trials, the pregnancy rate was less than 1 percent, and fertility returned to normal levels after users discontinued the device. The ParaGard, the other IUD product available in the United States, is a copper-bearing IUD that lasts ten years. Although the two types of devices have similar contraceptive efficacy and reversibility, users of the two different devices typically experience significantly different side effects. Whereas the copper T tends to increase menstrual bleeding and cramping, the levonorgestral-releasing IUD (LNG-IUD) reduces them. Clinical trials found that menstrual bleeding completely stops in 20 percent of Mirena users, a condition known as amenorrhea.

Several months after the Mirena insertion, I developed amenorrhea, which I embraced. As someone not particularly attached to menstruation as something that defines my femininity, I greatly appreciated not having to endure the inconveniences and physical discomfort that accompanied the monthly period. As an environmentalist, I was pleased not to have to produce any more tampon and sanitary napkin trash. This was a wonderfully liberating corporeal experience.[1] Mirena users who post their experience on the Internet often echo my sentiment. One thirty-five-year-old woman, for instance, wrote, "I LOVE my Mirena. . . . Mirena has made me feel free, not moody, no pain, no period."[2] Internet postings also reveal, however, that a significant number of women are experiencing undesirable side effects such as weight gain, mood swings, and loss of libido. These symptoms were not frequently observed in clinical trials but nevertheless are real and bothersome for these women.[3] Still other postings indicate that many women who are on Mirena after having tried other contraceptive methods are satisfied with the device. Sometimes Internet blogs mention the women's gynecologists, who are equally enthusiastic about this highly effective contraceptive. These doctors believe the device is safe and free of adverse side effects, and they view the altered menstrual pattern in a favorable light.

Mirena is marketed successfully within a pharmaceutical-marketing rubric of "lifestyle drugs." In other words, when a woman has a positive Mirena experience, the device is functioning as a pharmaceutical product that "promise[s] a refashioning of the material body with transformative life-enhancing results."[4] In recent years, pharmacological therapies claiming to treat baldness, sleep difficulties, excessive weight gain, mild depression, general aging, and sexual performance have become increasingly popular. These medications are not treatments for serious diseases. Rather, they treat or prevent various mild conditions that are often labeled a "problem." Taking a drug not only resolves the problem, but may also enhance the individual's life experience and productivity. For instance, low libido is now considered to be a health issue that can be fixed by medication for erectile dysfunction, which could simultaneously contribute to a man's overall well-being by increasing his sexual appetite, restoring what he perceives to be his manliness, and improving his outlook on life.[5] Similarly, decreased productivity at work might be treated with antidepressants, which are presumed to lift one's mood and help get through tasks more easily.[6]

Menstrual regulation and suppression medications that have become popular are yet another type of lifestyle drug. Feminist scholars Laura Mamo and Jennifer Fosket show that menstruation is cast as inconvenient, undesirable, and even unnatural in the marketing campaigns of Seasonale, the first oral contraceptive to reduce the number of menstrual periods from twelve to four a year. Various similar products are now being offered as a seemingly natural solution to what is sometimes viewed as a nagging female problem. By changing the material body, lifestyle drugs transform life from the inside out. Direct marketing to consumers of pharmaceutical products communicate this idea by presenting images of people whose lives are positively transformed by the medication.

When Mirena appeared on the TV screen around 2007, the commercial only briefly mentioned shorter, lighter periods as a common occurrence in users. Yet because the cultural narrative that renders menstrual suppression a positive lifestyle choice had already been solidified with period-reducing oral contraceptives, viewers were prepared to accept and appreciate the device's major side effect as a bodily enhancement. The advertisement, which shows a mother of three young boys appreciating her freedom from having to worry about birth control, conveys two additional ways the device improves women's lives through transforming the body. First, the ad suggests that the easy-to-use long-acting contraceptive enables a woman to "keep life simple." Second, it sends the message that retaining the option to have more children is another lifestyle choice that Mirena, a reversible method, allows a woman to make. To this end, the clip announces that the mother has "changed her mind" and concludes with a picture of her holding an adorable new baby girl standing with the rest of her happy upper-middle-class suburban white family.

To an average TV watcher, Mirena appears to be a new contraceptive product with unique features that promise to make a user's life better. The representation of the lifestyle IUD, however, obscures the history of the device and the broad spectrum of biopolitical interests that its development has engaged along the way. This chapter examines the making of Mirena, while revealing the behind-the-scenes aspects of this now increasingly popular contraceptive method and reconstructs the historical paths that produced this device. This activity, which I call *diffraction* after Donna Haraway's optical metaphor, shows how contemporary IUDs came to be, while simultaneously grasping the multiple meanings the device now embodies. The historical trajectories that made Mirena and the copper-bearing IUD ParaGard what they are today involved creating and reinforcing inequities among women of different races, classes, nationalities, ages, and levels of modernity. By tracking the backstories of how Mirena is represented, marketed, and embodied in the global North, this chapter brings into relief the transnational and racial political economies of women's bodies, health, and reproductive interests.

From a Population Control Tool to a Commercial Product

The period-free IUD that some of us love was created over the course of three decades. The first study to look at the effect of intrauterine administration of hormones was supported by the Ford Foundation and published in the journal *Fertility and Sterility* in 1970.[7] The Chicago researchers who inserted progesterone-releasing capsules into the womb observed changes in the uterine lining similar to those induced by oral contraceptives. They concluded that locally administering a hormonal substance in the uterus could be a way to increase the contraceptive effectiveness of IUDs.

Using discriminatory language common at the time to describe ideal IUD users, the authors related their study to the need for population control. According to them, women "in the less advanced countries" who lack "sophistication and motivation" were good candidates for this method because it achieves prolonged contraception "without special patient co-operation."[8] Early IUD studies presumed that women of the global South were not self-motivated to contracept, which justified the need for this new birth control method that could be imposed on women who, according to the population control advocates, were otherwise unwilling to limit their fertility or incapable of doing so. Studies of hormone-releasing IUDs initially drew their justification from a perceived need to increase reproductive control over former colonial subjects.

The primary goal of adding progesterone to an IUD was to decrease pregnancy rates of the existing plastic devices, which ranged from 2.3 to 10.8 per 100 women in one year. The researchers were pleased to find that no one wearing the progesterone-releasing device got pregnant during the study. The hormonal compound available at the time, however, lasted for only about twelve weeks, making the life span of the device "too short . . . to be meaningfully used in population control."[9] Nevertheless, the authors decided that what they had observed showed enough promise to suggest further development of this method.

The Next-Generation IUD

Research on hormone-releasing IUDs started at a time when developers were becoming frustrated with the performance of plastic IUDs. The effort to improve the inert devices by tinkering with their physical configurations seemed to take them nowhere. In the late 1960s, developers began investigating bioactive substances that could be added to IUDs to simultaneously increase contraceptive efficacy, reduce expulsion rates, and decrease bleeding and pain. The Population Council started developing copper-bearing devices with this intention in 1969. Other bioactive compounds such as estrogen and antiprogestin substances were also experimentally added to intrauterine devices, but these did not yield promising results.

This was also a time when the safety of the oral contraceptives was starting to be publicly questioned. It was becoming apparent that hormones from the oral contraceptive entering the bloodstream could cause severe headache, breast tenderness, and mood change, as well as rare but serious adverse consequences such as a fatal blood clot. This realization boosted the idea of administering hormones locally in the uterus, which theoretically would avoid systemic hormonal side effects. Within a few years, the authors of the 1970 study managed to develop a device that lasted six months. After testing it for twelve months, they concluded that its contraceptive effect was very good, although it needed to last longer for population management.[10] By the mid-1970s, a California-based company independently developed and started marketing a one-year progesterone-releasing IUD they called Progestasert, which stayed on the market on a small scale for the next couple of decades.[11]

The development of a multiyear hormone-releasing IUD, however, had to wait for the discovery of a synthetic progestin with high potency per unit weight that can be released slowly over many years. Such a compound emerged several years later from the Population Council's work to develop a hormone-releasing subdermal contraceptive implant. Sheldon Segal recounts his excitement when the idea of the "under-the-skin pill" came to him, and he experimentally implanted capsules filled with various hormones into rats in the council's laboratory.[12] Soon after, in 1970, the Population Council established the International Committee for Contraception Research (ICCR) to facilitate collaboration among a team of international scientists. The committee embarked on the development of the subdermal contraceptive with Elsimar Coutinho of Brazil as the head of the project.[13] After testing no fewer than ten compounds and a number of different capsules and rods, the research team selected levonorgestrel as the most promising progestin and ultimately produced the contraceptive method known as the Norplant.[14]

Another ICCR scientist, Tapani Luukkainen of Finland, led the development of the levonorgestrel-releasing IUD, and after more than a decade of testing to determine the appropriate dosage through a series of clinical trials, he introduced it in Finland in 1990 with the brand name Levonova.[15] Rebranded as Mirena in some other countries, the device was inserted in approximately 1 million women around the globe before it received approval from the U.S. Food and Drug Administration (FDA) in 2000 and started being sold to American women in 2001.

The Norplant Saga

Ironically, the Norplant, to which Mirena owed its hormonal compound, had been virtually withdrawn from the American market by 2001. The social reception of the Norplant after its introduction in the United States in 1990 was "mired in controversy, suspicion, and even ethnic conflicts" due to socially problematic applications of the device.[16] The idea of the under-the-skin pill was conceived when the Population Council was seeking a superior long-acting reversible contraceptive after it had come to realize that the IUD would not fulfill its expectation to become the one-size-fits-all solution for the problem of excess fertility in the global South. Norplant was in essence the next-generation imposable method and carried with it all of the problematic assumptions about controlling what the council saw as "excessively fertile" women's bodies. The biopolitical quality embedded in the implant technology was immediately expressed in the applications of Norplant in the United States. Within a few years, lawmakers proposed more than forty bills that either mandated Norplant use for women who received government assistance or targeted women who are poor, convicted, or addicted to drug and alcohol in order to prevent them from having children.[17] Norplant was also offered to poor inner-city adolescents at no cost in school-based clinics in Baltimore. The contraceptive implant was also distributed to the Native American population.[18] All of these applications were met with suspicion due to the "deep worries about discrimination in the United States on the basis of class, race, and gender."[19]

Some Norplant users also experienced undesirable and often unbearable hormonal side effects, including headache, acne, nausea, depression, scalp hair loss, weight gain, and irregular or heavy vaginal bleeding.[20] Yet these users could not easily discontinue the medication; they had to have a trained health care provider remove the Norplant, a painful procedure that involves making incisions in the arm, and often had to pay for this as well. Thousands of women filed lawsuits against its distributor, Wyeth-Ayerst Pharmaceuticals, claiming that the company failed to properly inform users about removal problems and adverse side effects. Most of the lawsuits were settled out of court or dismissed, and the company never lost a suit. Wyeth nevertheless suspended Norplant sales in the United States in 2000 after recalling a defective batch of the product and eventually withdrew the product completely from the American market.

Although Mirena is also a long-acting provider-dependent method using the same progestin as Norplant and both were developed by many of the same researchers, it has avoided being accused of discriminatory applications and becoming a target of concerted efforts to sue the provider. In part, Mirena has been helped by the timing of its release, which came after lessons were learned from the Norplant downfall. The Norplant controversy led to a public debate concerning moral and policy challenges of long-acting birth control methods. The Hastings Center, a nonpartisan research institute specializing in bioethics and public policy, assembled a task force that issued a report in 1995 on the ethics of long-term contraceptives.[21] Most members of the task force explicitly stated that compulsory use of contraceptives is unjustified for welfare recipients and generally in most other circumstances. Controversies and ethical debates around Norplant most likely discouraged lawmakers to recommend any new policies that involved long-term contraceptive methods. Mirena has thus far not become a target of public outrage, which has helped the device maintain a neutral image. The positive acceptance of Mirena also can be attributed to the fact that by 2001, the tragic incidents around the Dalkon Shield in the 1970s had been forgotten and a new generation of physicians and women was ready for a new contraceptive method.

Mirena's manufacturer has also kept a low profile, advertising the product in parenting magazines with images of content-looking well-to-do families and staying away from the population traditionally targeted in these problematic applications of imposable methods. In constructing an attractive product, the long-lasting effect of the device, which was problematized in the context of coerced contraception, has been recast as convenience with the assurance that the device can be removed if the woman changes her mind. The device's association with population control has been virtually wiped out by the clean and liberating image created by its TV commercial.

But this transformation did not occur automatically or overnight. Changes in the bleeding pattern caused by LNG-IUD took the device down a meandering path that necessitated sorting out the meaning of this side effect.

The Problem of Menstrual Bleeding

To discuss the issue of bleeding in IUD users, it is necessary to start back once again in the late 1960s when researchers admitted that they had failed to develop an ideal plastic device. They conceded that design innovation efforts focused too much on increasing the contraceptive efficacy and uterine retention and not enough on reducing side effects. Pain and bleeding resulted in so many discontinuations of the contraceptive method that the U.S. Agency for International Development (USAID) eventually decided to prioritize funding for research on a "bloodless, comfortable IUD."[22] Incidentally, the 1970 study had found that intrauterine hormone capsules decreased uterine contractions and vaginal bleeding. IUD researchers hence characterized progesterone as a "uterine tranquilizer" and hoped that future hormone-releasing IUDs would improve the overall efficacy of the contraceptive method by reducing cramping, pain, and bleeding.[23]

Although researchers knew these side effects were an obstacle to broader acceptance of IUDs, data to understand the problem in detail were scarce. Complaints of pain and discomfort were often characterized as psychological, and physicians dismissed them as a normal part of using the device for which certain women had low tolerance thresholds. The Cooperative Statistical Program (CSP), the multilocation large-scale statistical program that took place between 1963 and 1968 and validated the contraceptive efficacy of the IUD, reflects a lack of emphasis on women's subjective experiences. The study simply bundled "bleeding and/or pain" as a single category of reason for IUD removal.[24] It did not provide information on whether the patient requested removal because she could not tolerate menstrual cramping, had debilitating abdominal or back pain, experienced too much bleeding, found her period unacceptably prolonged, had too much midcycle spotting, or experienced some combination of symptoms. This made it impossible to analyze the relationship between side effects and removal in detail.

Because pain is difficult to measure objectively, systematic research on pain with IUD use is almost nonexistent. Blood loss, however, is quantifiable and is a source of health concern; hence, some researchers turned to measuring it in their studies. Studies found that, on average, women lose about 35 milliliters of blood during a menstrual period. Common plastic IUDs, which were larger in size and therefore more irritating to the uterus than smaller copper-bearing IUDs, increased the blood loss by 20 to 50 milliliters. The smaller copper-bearing IUDs increased blood loss by only 10 to 30 milliliters, although they prolonged the period by two days. The particular progesterone-releasing devices being tested decreased blood loss by 40 percent.[25] Although no research had confirmed that IUDs could cause anemia, developers suggested that increased menstrual bleeding might cause the health of poor women of the global South to decline since approximately half of them already had anemia or were borderline anemic. These data raised some hope in the minds of researchers that hormone-releasing IUDs might be distributed to women of the global South as protection against anemia.[26]

The Cultural Significance of Menstruation

In the meantime, IUD developers also began to notice that dropout rates of subjects from their studies who complained of bleeding and pain varied dramatically from place to place. A 1970 study of 14,000 users in thirty countries found that removal due to bleeding and pain was relatively rare in Europe. Yet they found significant variance in the global South. Parts of India, for example, had a much higher incidence of dropouts from studies compared to other parts of the country, whereas incidents in the Philippines were much lower.[27]

These findings prompted the Population Council to sponsor another study, this one investigating the effect of culture on IUD acceptance. Elizabeth Whelan reported that Orthodox Jewish women were five times more likely than non-Orthodox Jewish women to discontinue the IUD on account of prolonged or irregular bleeding because their religious practice mandated that women refrain from various religious, daily, and sexual activities during their period. She also identified religious texts that could have similar effects on women of other faiths.[28] Subsequently the 1979 *Population Reports,* which summarized the status of IUD research for family planning programmers and other health professionals, stated: "In countries where menstruating women are not permitted to prepare certain foods, carry on their usual household tasks, perform religious rites, or engage in sexual intercourse, any prolongation of bleeding or midcycle spotting disrupts personal and household routines. As a result, not only the IUD user but also her husband and mother-in-law may insist on removal of the device."[29] This shows that users' cultural beliefs began to be seen as part of the problem that led to the discontinuation of IUDs.

As an organization overseeing reproductive health around the globe, the World Health Organization (WHO) also recognized that menstrual disturbances, such as no bleeding, excessive bleeding, or irregular bleeding, were responsible for one-fourth to one-half of all first-year dropouts of contraceptive methods such as the IUD, progestin-only oral contraceptive, progestin-estrogen combination pill, and progesterone injection. Between 1973 and 1979, the WHO conducted an investigation of attitudes toward menstruation among 5,000 women from fourteen cultures.[30] Interviews with women affirmed that an increase in the number of bleeding days might be unacceptable in certain cultures because it interferes with day-to-day household or religious activities. Three-quarters of the Hindu women interviewed, for instance, said they avoided cooking for their families during menstruation; almost all respondents in Egypt, Indonesia, and Pakistan and three-quarters of Yugoslavian Muslim women believed that a woman should not visit temples when she is bleeding. The study also found that while many women felt that increased blood loss would make them physically weaker, some also believed that decreased blood loss would cause discomfort due to retention of blood within the body. Importantly, the study concluded that most women did not want any changes in their menstrual patterns.

As the WHO report was coming out, the Population Council discovered that its latest levonorgestrel-releasing device was experiencing a 20 percent discontinuation rate due to amenorrhea or other hormonal side effects.[31] At this early phase in the testing of the device, researchers had not understood that levonorgestrel stopped menstrual bleeding altogether in 20 percent of users. The initial high dropout rate therefore was later attributed to uninformed physicians who removed the device out of concern that was actually unwarranted. But this explanation provided only a small consolation since the WHO study had also found that the majority of women interviewed stated that they were "not prepared to accept" a contraceptive if it led to amenorrhea.[32] The rates of women rejecting amenorrhea varied from 53 percent of British women to 91 percent of Punjab women in Pakistan, while their reasons ranged from fear of impairing their health by disallowing what they viewed as "bad blood" to purge and reluctance to tamper with nature to the negative indications of menopause and infertility associated with having no periods.

Defying the original expectation that reduced blood loss and less cramping with progesterone-releasing devices would increase IUD acceptance in the global South, the 1982 *Population Reports* concluded that removal rates in several trials were similar to or worse for the hormone-releasing devices as compared to the copper-bearing ones.[33] Although levonorgestrel had achieved the "bloodless, comfortable IUD" sought by USAID, the cultural significance of menstruation appeared to be working against the acceptance of an otherwise effective device. As this perception unfolded, the conceptual division between users of the global North and South widened.

Configuring the Modern Woman/Consumer

The WHO study also offered subtle yet significant insight into who may be more inclined to accept modern contraceptive methods that alter menstrual patterns. For instance, the report noted that beliefs associated with menstruation, such as that one should not bathe or visit the temple while bleeding, were more commonly held by "older, less educated, rural women." In contrast, a woman who was "prepared to accept" amenorrhea was reportedly "younger, better educated, [and] urban."[34] Family planning in the global South has been closely linked to the idea of modernity representing enlightenment values of secularism, rationality, scientism, and optimism for the future. As Nilanjana Chatterjee and Nancy Riley point out, the modern subject has been construed as a rational, autonomous individual who can control her environment and shape her own future by embracing scientific knowledge and technological innovations.[35] As researchers took notice of the cultural significance of menstrual disturbance, however, they began to see that some women who lacked education and led a preindustrial lifestyle were not modern enough to accept scientific methods of fertility control that change bleeding patterns.

The presumed unpreparedness of women of the global South to accept the new contraceptive was compounded by the way clinical studies in the region were interpreted and represented. An Indian study comparing the copper-bearing to the levonorgestrel-releasing device found that the continuation rate of the latter was significantly lower due to amenorrhea and irregular bleeding.[36] The seven-year study initiated by the Population Council, which took place mostly in clinics located in the global South, including Brazil, Egypt, Chile, the Dominican Republic, Brazil, and Singapore, also showed a better continuation rate for the copper-bearing device.[37] The double-blind test protocols that prevented physicians from providing adequate counseling about amenorrhea may have increased the number of removals in these trials. But this background was obscured when the 1995

Population Reports simply noted that LNG-IUD removal rates were higher than copper-bearing IUDs in the global South due to amenorrhea.[38] The report left the impression that LNG-IUD was not well suited for women in underdeveloped areas who embody premodern ideas about menstruation.

The *Population Reports* then presented a contrasting conclusion from a European study, which had resulted in less common discontinuation for bleeding and pain with the LNG-IUD than with the copper IUD.[39] The comparable success of the LNG-IUDs in the European study conducted in Denmark, Finland, Hungary, Norway, and Sweden was attributed to having provided detailed information regarding the contraceptive method to the women who received it. Health care personnel in the European trial explained to their patients how the effect of the hormone reduces the buildup of the uterine lining that sheds during menstruation. They also informed them that amenorrhea is not a sign of pregnancy or menopause, that the ovarian function is continuing even in the absence of menstruation, and that amenorrhea does not reduce the ability to conceive after removing the device. In addition, Scandinavian women were told that the LNG-IUD had a high level of effectiveness, which motivated them to continue using the method. Some were also advised of the device's benefits, such as increased hemoglobin, better iron stores, general well-being, and relief from dysmenorrhea and prolonged bleeding. Information regarding what women should expect to experience with this device as well as its health benefits were also disseminated through mass media. Tapani Luukkainen, whose name is often associated with the invention of LNG-IUDs, explains that offering open and accurate information has contributed to the acceptance of this method of contraception.[40]

Based on the positive responses in Europe, Luukkainen announced: "When adequately advised beforehand, most women who develop amenorrhea learn to like the new freedom."[41] This seemingly nonproblematic statement fails to recognize that a medicalized explanation of the female reproductive system may have resonated with the women in the European study due to their cultural upbringing. Medical anthropologist Emily Martin has found that middle-class American women more readily identified with the scientific model of menstruation as compared to working-class women, who resisted medical explanations of their embodied experiences.[42] Martin's findings suggest that certain groups of women are more amenable to seeing their bodies in physiological terms, making them good candidates for accepting the information of the hormonal effects on their reproductive systems. Luukkainen does not address how "adequate advising" may work for women whose understanding of their bodies departs significantly from the medicalized version. His suggestion to educate women may certainly be effective for the middle class of the global North but does not necessarily take all women into consideration. In fact, as Stacy Pigg points out, knowledge of bodies is always cultural and there exists no neutral biological language that is equivalent across cultures. Insisting on Western scientific understandings of reproduction thus could constitute "epistemological colonization" or violence.[43]

Writing Off Less Modern Women

After the comparative clinical trials in the global South showed a lower retention rate for hormonal devices, there has been little attempt to see if acceptance by these women could be improved if they were "adequately advised." In fact, interest in women who were not ready to accept amenorrhea faded as researchers turned their attention to women who might "learn to like" the period-less lifestyle. If there are indeed health benefits of this device, such advantages are being denied to women of the global South, who are implicitly written off as being not modern enough to appreciate the new technology.

Perhaps IUD developers have simply lost interest in women who they deem as less modern. But there is also little incentive for family planning supporters to strongly promote the distribution of this device overseas, now that the copper-bearing devices are widely accepted. This is particularly so since they are just as effective in preventing pregnancy and are much more economical. When asked whether USAID would provide Mirena to overseas family planning programs, Dr. James D. Shelton, senior medical scientist of the agency's Office of Population, gave this answer on his Q&A Web site, *Jim Shelton's Pearls*: "Cost is likely to be an insurmountable hurdle. . . . Bear in mind, the Copper-T-380A is an excellent and inexpensive IUD. So after factoring in the costs of introducing a new method, the advantages of Mirena would only justify USAID large-scale procurement in the face of a very attractive price."[44] This statement construes Mirena as being too expensive for aid agencies to supply to women in the global South because the copper T is an adequate cheaper alternative.

In order to close some of the economic gap, the Population Council and Mirena manufacturer Schering Oy established the International Contraceptive Access Foundation (ICA) in 2004. ICA offers a combination of donation and subsidized sale (for a maximum of $40 per device) to the public sector for a limited number of units. The ICA also conducts projects in twelve countries supporting Mirena use in family planning programs.[45] Nevertheless, the $40 price tag is still vastly more expensive than the $1.64 that USAID supplies the copper T for. Copper IUDs can actually be obtained as cheaply as $0.25 a unit.[46] The economic factor clearly widens the gulf between the reproductive choices of women in the global North and South.

The economic divide is present in the United States as well. Mirena costs around $500 at a doctor's office, compared to about $250 for ParaGard, in addition to the office visit charges and fees for screening tests.[47] State Medicaid programs may cover Mirena at various levels of reimbursement, and an uninsured patient whose income is below the poverty level can apply for a free device with her provider through a program funded by Bayer HealthCare Pharmaceuticals.[48] More often than not, however, women must cover all or part of the expense. Paradoxically, despite the high initial cost, IUDs, including the Mirena, are the most cost-effective form of reversible contraception.[49]

As ideas formulated regarding who would accept a device that dramatically changes menstrual patterns, who could be educated to appreciate decreased menstrual bleeding, and who could afford the high initial expenses, the original intention to promote the hormone-releasing IUD in the global South to boost contraceptive acceptance evaporated. Developers instead found new interest in applying the device's unique side effect to gynecological treatments, as we shall see next. Looking at these ironic transitions teaches us a few things: biopolitical investments in women's bodies diverge over space and time; developers transfer their interests from one type of device application to another without explicit reflections on how they perpetuate inequality; and technological practices are imagined with implicit assumptions about differences between women of the global South and North. Significantly, shifting interests kept the momentum for the exploration of hormone-releasing devices.

A Contraceptive with Therapeutic Properties

One such interest was the idea of turning the hormone-releasing IUD into a therapeutic device. When the original progesterone-releasing devices were found to decrease menstrual blood loss by 40 percent, researchers toyed with the idea of using hormonal IUDs to treat or prevent anemia. Applying the device to anemia was a logical extension of their initial goal to improve the method's acceptance in the global South: the device would be more attractive if it could be argued that it had additional health benefits for the population. To this end, the ICCR conducted a study in the Dominican Republic in the late 1980s and found that the LNG-IUD appears to reduce the proportion of women with clinical anemia and improve their iron level.[50] Researchers concluded that the device might become a strong health-enhancing tool since it both prevents pregnancy, which depletes women's energy, and decreases blood loss that leads to anemia. In other words, investigation into applying the device for the improvement of women's health was initiated in relationship to a disease that is more prevalent in the global South. Applications to other gynecological conditions, however, quickly took over.

In a 1995 article, Tapani Luukkainen and Juhani Toivonen reconceptualized the levonorgestrel-IUD as a contraceptive with "therapeutic properties."[51] They reported that the LNG-IUD dramatically improved the conditions of women who suffered excessive menstrual bleeding, a condition called menorrhagia, and that the device might offer an alternative for surgical treatments such as hysterectomy and endometrial ablation (destroying of the uterine lining). They introduced findings that showed the LNG-IUD reduces endometrial hyperplasia, or the excess growth of the uterine lining, which occasionally leads to uterine cancer. They announced that these "promising findings" warrant further investigations into the use of the device to treat this problem.[52] They also reported that some observations suggested that long-time use of the device reduced the incidence of uterine fibroids (benign uterine tumors that can cause painful periods, back pain, and sometimes infertility). And they added that the LNG-IUD could also be used to prevent the endometrium from cancerous growth in women who are taking estrogen to manage menopausal symptoms.

Luukkainen's enthusiasm was amplified ten years later, in 2005, at the Fifth International Symposium on the Intrauterine Devices and Systems for Women's Health sponsored by the Population Council and the United Nations Population Fund, which I attended. Nearly half of the presentations focused on the levonorgestrel intrauterine system, many of them discussing experiences or the possibilities of applying the device to treatment or prevention of gynecological conditions. Illnesses mentioned included menorrhagia, dysmenorrhea (menstruation accompanied by severe pain), endometrial hyperplasia, endometriosis (uterine-lining-like tissue growing outside the uterus, which can cause debilitating pelvic pain and can also cause internal organs to fuse together), adenomyosis (uterine lining tissue that grows inside the muscular wall of the uterus, causing pain), uterine fibroids, uterine polyps, and endometrial carcinoma (uterine cancer).[53] The possibility of seeking FDA approval to prescribe the device as the progestin component of hormone replacement therapy for menopausal women was also discussed.[54] Overall, the researchers were excited about conducting more studies and the possibility of their device's being offered as an alternative treatment to surgery or oral progestin treatments for many gynecological disorders. Incidentally, Mirena received FDA approval in early 2010 for the treatment of menorrhagia.

The growing interest in the therapeutic use of the LNG-IUD further steered its researchers away from their initial neo-Malthusian intentions to distribute the device to women in the global South. Preventing or healing disease and maintaining the health of their own patients as well as encouraging their colleagues to adopt this new technique, have instead become the new biopolitical interest for Mirena researchers.

The Biopolitical Script of Menstrual Suppression Technologies

Surpassing the device's promise for the diseased patients is the appeal that device-induced menstrual pattern changes has for general consumers. Contraceptives that are approved as menstrual management methods have paved the way for Mirena to be perceived as having a similar benefit. Less apparent is the fact that the histories of these medications are intimately linked to the development of the LNG-IUD with overlapping researchers.

Is Menstruation Obsolete?

Contraceptive developers were paying attention to altered menstrual patterns before they became an issue for IUD users. During the 1950s, Gregory Pincus, the inventor of the first oral contraceptive, noticed that his trial subjects became distressed when they experienced amenorrhea, which led him to believe that women wanted to feel that they were menstruating naturally. Then the director of biological research of G. D. Searle, the first company to market oral contraceptives, told Pincus that he "did not want to take part in the development of any compound that might interfere with the menstrual cycle."[55] In response, Pincus devised a way of mimicking nature by creating the seven-day bleeding period every twenty-one days, which is actually caused by taking sugar pills for a week instead of hormones.[56] The inventors of the oral contraceptive thus effectively configured a woman whose "normal" periods consist of a twenty-eight-day menstrual cycle twelve times a year.

Forty years later, contraceptive researchers started to reconfigure the menstruating subject. After decades of experience with contraceptive methods that inadvertently affected menstrual patterns, Elsimar Coutinho and Sheldon Segal, who were involved in the development of both the Norplant and the LNG-IUD, published *Is Menstruation Obsolete?* Their 1999 book contends that menstruation is "an unnecessary, avoidable byproduct of the human reproductive process."[57] The authors state that regular and recurrent menstruation throughout most of a woman's fertile years is a fairly recent phenomenon of the industrialized world: women used to have very few periods when they nursed babies for an extended period of time and gave birth multiple times throughout their reproductive lives. The authors argue that the common perception that menstruation is a natural event that is somehow beneficial to women has no scientific basis.

Since there were no products indicated for menstrual suppression on the market yet, Coutinho and Segal proposed that women should start using available methods to stop menstruation "with the cooperation and supervision of their physicians."[58] This could be done, for instance, by skipping the sugar pills in standard oral contraceptives. The authors predicted that suppressing menstruation "would forge a major advance in women's health, led by women" and that "today's proposal would become tomorrow's new paradigm."[59] Subscribing to the idea that biological differences hold women down and proposing to liberate them from their innate imperative, the authors quoted the most prominent birth control activist of all times, ending the book by stating, "The pioneer feminist Margaret Sanger wrote 'No woman is completely free unless she has control over her own reproductive system.' Let this new freedom begin."[60] Their prediction about the new paradigm has for the most part come true. Although pharmaceutical companies, instead of women, led the way with their new products, the idea that a woman could suppress her menstruation to free herself from an unnecessary burden has taken hold among consumers in North America and Europe.

Marketing Menstrual Suppression Products

Laura Mamo and Jennifer Fosket illustrate how Seasonale, an oral contraceptive that produces menses-like bleeding cycles four times a year, rewrote the norms of menstruation and menstruating subjects through its product campaign. In the absence of either pathology or an at-risk state that requires medication, the Seasonale campaign constructed menstruation as an inconvenience and an obstacle that the drug could eliminate. It told women, "There is no medical reason to have [a period] when you are on the pill," suggesting that since the periods that pill users experience are in effect created by the medication, reducing the frequency of unnatural periods is perfectly reasonable.[61] Its marketing discourse also "produced associations between cleanliness and femininity, between freedom of movement and women's bodies, and between limited menstrual flow and natural embodiment," thereby reconfiguring the nonmenstruating woman as desirable and feminine.[62]

Since the launch of Seasonale by Duramed Pharmaceuticals in 2003, a number of similar products have been introduced. Seasonique from Duramed also induces menstrual-like bleeding every three months. The TV commercial for this product shows a physician, who announces, "There is no medical need to have a monthly period on the pill. Lots of women are having four periods a year." Based on what she learned from the doctor, a young woman in the ad decides to use the drug, conveying to the viewers that such a decision is a logical one. A rival product, Loestrin 24 Fe from Warner Chilcott, reduces monthly bleeding to three days or less. This product is marketed with a catchphrase, "Say so long to a period that's too long." Its advertisement features Cammie, a young, active, and attractive woman living in an artsy neighborhood in New York City.

Suggestive scenes of a bouquet of red roses and of a man's arm around her waist send the message that the drug produces an appealing heterosexual female body that is available for sex for more days each month. Finally, the most recent product, Lybrel from Wyeth Pharmaceuticals (now Pfizer), eliminates bleeding entirely within about six months by continuously taking progestin-estrogen combination birth control pills. As with other lifestyle drugs, modifying the material body with menstrual suppression products produces culturally and socially meaningful positive changes in the identities and lives of their users.

Mirena's Additional Benefit and Governmentality

Mirena is not explicitly marketed as a menstrual regulation product. Yet some of its informational material, such as the pamphlet provided to prescribing physicians, highlights the side effect as an "additional benefit."[63] The 2006 educational DVD for patients also promotes this aspect with an illustrative episode of an apparently athletic career-oriented woman, who recommends Mirena to her sister because she likes not having her period. The 2008 TV commercial, which introduced the product widely to prospective consumers, merely mentions a "shorter lighter period" as a common side effect. Yet since many women are already familiar with menstrual-suppression contraceptives, they are likely to interpret reduced bleeding as a bonus feature.

Women who blog about how much they love Mirena regularly attribute their satisfaction to their nonmenstruating bodies as much as they do to not having to worry about forgetting to take the pill.[64] The precedence of menstrual-suppression medications prepared Mirena users to view their experience with the device as an enhancement of lifestyle. These commercial products have reconfigured menstruation and the menstruating subjects, successfully transforming the meaning of monthly periods from a necessary part of womanly embodiment to an event that can be manipulated to suit one's lifestyle.

A biopolitical script based on market logic and capitalist lifestyle has been co-configured into menstrual-suppressing contraceptives. As Patrick Joyce points out, the emergence of liberalism in Europe "depended on cultivating a certain sort of self, one that was reflexive and self-watching."[65] The enlightened women who make conscious decisions about how they are going to manage their reproductive lives and maximize their bodily functions to live life smartly and productively are *ruled through freedom*. The marketing of this lifestyle drug relies on self-governing subjects whose desires are cultivated through the advertising, who exercise their right to manage their own fertility, and who choose to maintain their reproductive health. In the context of the American market, the biopolitical subjects of the long-acting menstrual-free IUD are largely invested in as a site of consumption rather than as an overtly fertile population. They are the subjects of liberal governmentality. A closer investigation of how IUD users are represented in product promotional materials, however, offers additional insight into how governance over women's bodies is delicately differentiated at intersections of race and class.

The Racial Economy of IUD Promotion in the United States

Marketing endorsements of IUDs today argue that the contraceptive method has advantages over the pill and barrier methods because it has long-term effectiveness that offers convenience and a lower rate of user failure. They also promote it as being favorable compared to surgical sterilization: the device's contraceptive effect is reversible, and it preserves future fertility. Not all women's reproductive choices, however, are represented equally in the advertisements. The device's benefits tend to be advertised through representations of women who are subtly differentiated in accordance with cultural expectations about how certain groups of women should regulate their reproductive capacities. While the construction of the North/South divide in IUD applications reflected ideas about modernity based on regionalized racialization and economics, promotional materials for the devices within the United States reveal that biopolitical interests are segmented based on race and class, mirroring American social relations.

Terri Kapsalis makes a similar observation in a three-page Norplant advertisement printed in a nurse practitioner's journal in 1992, arguing that they implicitly reinforce race-based reproductive politics.[66] Both of the two white women featured in the ad have children and appear modern, wealthy, and family oriented. The first woman chose Norplant because she is mostly certain that she completed her family but would like to leave open the option of having more children, while the second one is using the implant to time the birth of the next child she plans to have. Both are photographed with their children. The African American woman in the advertisement, in contrast, has no children. Rather, she is using Norplant so that she can finish nursing school before she has a family. Kapsalis points out that the representation of the childless African American woman reflects the idea that a black woman should establish herself economically before she has children and signals that Norplant will aid this process. She argues that these advertisement images and narratives "play into current dominant constructions of proper African American women's reproductive identity."[67] I would add that a strong expectation toward family orientedness in white women is also embedded in these advertisements.

Subtle but racially distinct similar messages are present in the marketing of IUDs. Of the two products available in the United States, the ParaGard Web site shows far more diversity than the Mirena site.[68] Women represented on the Mirena site are mostly upper-middle-class white women with their male partners and children; only one light-skinned African American woman can be found posing with her even lighter-skinned baby girl, but without a male partner, in a tastefully decorated nursery.[69] One can deduce that the primary target niche market for this product is well-to-do mothers.

In comparison, ParaGard reaches out to a broader consumer base, including women who have not had children. The product home page features five racially diverse women. With a scroll of the mouse, the viewer can read the reason each woman chose ParaGard. The Asian woman, who is "single and planning for the future," is "in a serious relationship, but not ready for a family." She represents a woman of color who is expected to establish her livelihood before she has children. The race of the woman in a business suit standing confidently in the center can be read as either a dark-haired white person or a very light-skinned Latina. She represents a career-oriented woman who wants to put off having a family. One of the African American women appeals to prospective users who are "concerned about hormonal health risks" and want "highly effective birth control" without hormones and their side effects. The other African American woman is "living the change of life" and represents older consumers. Her testimony reads: "Done with family. Done with pills, patches, and rings. Wants simple birth control to last until menopause." Whereas the Asian and Latina/white women clearly express the desire to have children in the future, the two African American women do not. The second woman explicitly states her childbearing is complete, and the first woman makes no mention of wanting a child.

African American women's desire to restrain their fertility is a culturally appropriate script that is also played out in the representation of Mirena users. The Mirena patient education DVD features women of color in only one of the four episodes: two African American women discuss Mirena as a good option for them because their chaotic lives with children make it challenging to remember to take the pill. One of them (whose feature can also be read as a non–African American woman of color) is pregnant with her second child and asks her gynecologist if Mirena is right for her; the white female doctor assures her that it is not too early to plan on getting it during her postnatal checkups. An ideal user for Mirena as represented in this episode reiterates the notion that the IUD is a suitable contraceptive for women who are unreliable pill users (who are often marked by their race, class, and young age) and for restraining the fertility of women of color.

The three educational DVD episodes involving white women include the one I have already mentioned, which features an athletic businesswoman who appreciates not having her period. The second skit shows a new mom with her husband. She wishes she did not have to fiddle with the diaphragm whenever the couple finally has a moment to themselves. Sure enough, her doctor recommends Mirena. This scenario highlights the sexual spontaneity and convenience that Mirena users in a stable relationship enjoy. The last episode presents a blond white woman with three children. She says she considered tubal ligation, but decided to get a Mirena instead because she is not completely sure if she is done having children.

There is a striking similarity between this woman and the fifth woman shown on the ParaGard Web site. She is also a blond white woman, who "loves being a mom." With a scroll of the mouse, we learn that she "adores her kids. Wonders what it would be like to have more. Wants hassle-free birth control that won't limit her options." The Mirena TV commercial also emphasizes reversibility as an advantage of this contraceptive method, concluding the clip with a picture-perfect American family with their fourth newborn child. But with a closer and critical look, this so-called option is presented as appropriate only for middle- to upper-middle-class white family-oriented mothers. There is an enduring pattern that shows a cultural preference toward fecund women to be portrayed as white and well-to-do and toward women of color to express the need to suppress reproduction.

In an essay titled "Will the 'Real' Mother Please Stand Up?: The Logic of Eugenics and American National Family Planning," Patricia Hill Collins argues that in the United States, "where social class, race, ethnicity, gender, sexuality, and nationality comprise intersecting dimensions of oppression, not all mothers are created equal."[70] The idealized mother best suited for the tasks of reproducing both the American nation and seemingly American values is embodied by an affluent white woman bearing American citizenship who reproduces her biological children and physically participates in every facet of their lives. These kinds of mothers, whom Collins calls "real" mothers, encounter social policies, institutional arrangements, and ideological messages that encourage and support them to continue to reproduce. For instance, the availability of medical services to combat infertility simultaneously supports and obligates upper-middle-class white women to reproduce their biological offspring. Images of large, happy families with distinctly white upper-middle-class features such as the ones shown on IUD commercials are examples of the encouragement that "real" mothers receive. In contrast, mothers who are considered less fit and even unfit are discouraged from having children and do not receive similar support for parenting. The reproductive options that are prescribed to working-class black women, in particular, often derive from the racist notion of poor African American women who have too many children and become "welfare queens." Collins argues that both positive and negative eugenics, which are based on the race and class of the mothers, are still present in contemporary American society. We indeed see them manifest in contraceptive advertisements.

On the surface, ParaGard and Mirena IUDs have joined the myriad birth control options available to American consumers. Yet various aspects of the contraceptive method are matched up with culturally sanctioned body/technology relationships. Although sometimes bodies cross over the dichotomous categories, reversibility is generally stressed for what are viewed as real American mothers, and other aspects, such as the ease of use and long-term effectiveness, are promoted through the bodies of women of color. The initial emphases IUD researchers placed on controlling the birthrates of undesirable populations and disciplining women's bodies to suppress socially problematic pregnancies are still embodied by this seemingly progressive lifestyle product.

Body/Technology Relationships in Racialized Global Contexts

During its fifty years of development, the IUD discourse has generated diverse body/technology relationships while representing scientific findings in biopolitically and geopolitically meaningful ways. From being the population control tool it once was foreseen to become, the hormone-releasing device diversified into a gynecological treatment, a menstrual-suppression technique, and an alternative to tubal ligation. The diversification, however, applies for the most part only to the global North. The International Contraceptive Access Foundation, an organization that donates free LNG-IUDs to family programs overseas, states, "ICA aims to serve the needs of women and families in the developing world to achieve their desired family size and birth spacing."[71] As this statement suggests, the biopolitics of contraceptive technologies in the global South continue to focus on fertility, although the rhetoric has moved away from justifying mass insertions. The pairing of excessively fertile bodies and an effective long-acting contraceptive technology remains the dominant paradigm there.

Contested meanings of menstruation have contributed to reinforcing the divide between bodies in the global South and North by creating an additional dichotomy between "backward" and "modern" contraceptive users. Women who were deemed not ready to appreciate amenorrhea due to their cultural beliefs about menstruation were left behind in the popularization of the hormone-releasing device. Meanwhile, those regarded as accepting of the scientific explanation of why women should embrace less menstrual bleeding were thrust into a new paradigm of bodily enhancement and lifestyle medications. The cost of Mirena, too, has contributed to the separation between underprivileged women, for whom effective contraceptives are rendered adequate, and economically privileged women, for whom a favorable contraceptive should offer extra benefits.

As Mirena's common side effect acquired new meanings, body/technology relationships in the global North expanded. IUD developers interested in treating menstrual disorders and uterine ailments reconceptualized the device as a therapeutic technology and gynecological patients as treatable bodies. Much less concerned with reproduction, this body/technology coupling represents the biopolitics of health maintenance. The menses-free body/device also entered a market already sold on the idea of artificial menstrual suppression as lifestyle choice. Liberal governmentality or self-management for achieving better health, higher productivity, and a happier life connects the desiring consumer to this new contraceptive with an additional benefit.

The latest body/technology relationships in IUD promotional materials also represent contemporary eugenics ideologies promoted within the framework of individualism. The 1995 Hastings Center Report on the ethics of long-acting contraceptives signify a shift in the approach to suppressing undesirable pregnancies from targeting specific groups to holding individuals responsible. Authors of the report take great caution not to approve of broad use that may suggest racial and class discrimination. Yet at the same time they explore acceptable ways to discourage what they see as irresponsible reproduction. The overall report leaves an opening for an argument to be made for promoting long-acting contraceptive methods in limited cases that are evaluated on an individual basis. The individualist approach easily blends with a consumerist framework and naturalizes the coupling of racialized bodies, understood as potentially "unfit mothers," with long-acting and user-failure-free contraceptives. Meanwhile, white mothers' bodies are unproblematically paired with the reversible feature of the IUD, implicitly promoting positive eugenics through consumption.

By following the development of Mirena, this chapter traced how diverse biopolitical subjects were constructed within the IUD discourse in accordance with cultural expectations about race and class, as well as the global political economy of women's bodies that render some as overproducing fertility machines and others as sites of consumption of medical services and devices. It also revealed how various body/technology pairings were configured, forming a network of relationships that reflect the racialized global context within which technoscientific interventions in women's bodies are imagined.

6   Diffracting the Technoscientific Body: A Conclusion

Discourses are not just "words"; they are material-semiotic practices through which objects of attention and knowing subjects are both constituted.

Diffraction patterns record the history of interaction, interference, reinforcement, difference.

—Donna Haraway[1]

Throughout this book, I have traced the making of a politically versatile technology—a device readily appropriated by diverse social agendas ranging from population control to the antiabortion movement. The optical metaphor of diffraction is the methodological tool I used to tease out the biopolitical scripts embodied by the IUD. Each chapter analyzed different diffraction patterns created by a particular interference I chose to make in the history of the device's development. Chapter 2 detailed the Population Council's quest to fashion a birth control plan for a nation. Diffracting the device in this instance illuminated the colonial legacy of the scientific domination over native women's bodies and shed light on the material-discursive construction of the population control device. Chapter 3 focused on the changing concept of risk to illustrate how the users who were considered "ideal" were transformed from the masses to moms. While examining the development of the copper T against the shifting receptions of the IUD in the United States and internationally, diffractive patterns in this chapter showed how biopolitical scripts of the device diversified over the years.

   Chapter 4 concentrated on the two contesting views on the IUD's mechanism of action, revealing how opposing theories of the contraceptive mechanism have been constructed, buttressed, and challenged. It elucidated how the antichoice politics managed to penetrate the IUD discourse despite resistance from IUD developers who support the pro-choice feminist agenda. Chapter 5 used the hormone-releasing device to track the manifestations of body/technology relationships that reinforce global racial and class hierarchies. This was done by diffracting the high-end consumer product Mirena, following its research and development trajectories over the past forty years. Each chapter began its story by returning to the 1960s when the IUD was first conceptualized as a population control tool to show that differently configured devices have their roots in an imposable device.

In short, diffractive methodology enabled me to parse out the heterogeneous constructions of implicated users, their bodies, and modes of governance that are intertwined and embedded in a single category of devices: the IUD. It is now time to summarize the key findings and consider how feminists might engage with the heterogeneity of meanings inherent in politically versatile technologies and build a multidimensional movement that supports progressive agendas.

Appropriating Women in the Scientific Discourse

A significant aspect of my investigation focused on how diverse political interests in women's bodies became incorporated into the knowledge production processes of contraceptive development. This study showed that a key mechanism behind the making of this politically versatile technology involved emphasizing the differences among women whenever it helped to achieve cultural acceptance for the IUD. In the process, some women were deemed individual agents of contraceptive choice, while others were denied agency. Another essential process entailed effacing the differences among women, which enabled the creation of a universally applicable technology. Combining the two mechanisms enabled the production of this heterogeneous yet seemingly singular artifact.

In asserting the differences among women, a paradigmatic distinction between "Western individuals" and the "population" was made first and foremost. Women in the global South were conceptualized in the aggregate as the population, and their bodies were seen as reproductive machines, the output of which (i.e., the number of offspring) needed to be regulated. The perceived urgent need to control women's bodies in order to set a nation on its path to modernity supported the development of an imposable contraceptive method that would be distinct from birth control methods that rely on the individuals to use them effectively and methodically. Throughout the years, the notion of a user-failure-free method kept resurfacing, along with new constructions of users whose fertility must be suppressed. They included the domestic masses on welfare, irresponsible teenagers, and racial minorities who should establish their economic means before having children. The IUD discourse stripped these women of the global South and underprivileged women of the global North of their personal agencies, constantly differentiating them from women with racial, economic, and citizen-based privileges.

A variety of implicated users were opportunistically constructed in the IUD discourse as certain types of consumers of the global North, who were often demarcated from the masses and the population. Constructions of "individual" users more often than not helped bolster the favorability of the IUD as a contraceptive device. For instance, the monogamous mother with a "safe" body helped restore confidence in the copper T as an acceptable contraceptive method after the reputation of the IUD was ruined by the Dalkon Shield crisis in the United States. Similarly, the so-called progressive woman who prefers less menstrual bleeding boosted the feasibility of the hormone-releasing device as a consumer product. Configurations of these users who were considered ideal also involved the construction of users who were considered inappropriate. As opposed to mothers, who presumably were less prone to sexually transmitted infections due to their monogamous sexual relations and were less likely to sue a provider should they experience difficulty in conceiving children after IUD use, childless young women were assumed to be promiscuous, litigious, and too risky to receive this contraceptive method. In the making of the period-free device, women of the global South were regarded as users who held backward views on menstruation and could not afford expensive devices. The so-called conservative religious woman was constructed by the antiabortion discourse as a refuser of IUDs. In all cases, differences among women were emphasized to conceptualize a particular application of the device.

Unlike the "population" or the implicated user of the imposable device whose agency was denied, "individual" users were conceptualized as agents who would choose (or refuse) the IUD as a method of contraception. Whereas the imposable device governed users' bodies simply by occupying the uterus and preventing pregnancy, modes of governance over individual bodies were variously tailored to uphold a particular configuration of the technology. In order to maintain the safety of the copper T, prospective users were carefully screened in the United States to make sure they were good candidates. Mirena users were expected to appreciate the menstrual-free lifestyle and use the device to free them to keep up with the demands of motherhood, family, and profession. Religious women were directed to view their bodies as potential sites of sin and the IUD as an abortifacient and to refuse to accept the device. All of these co-configurations of technology, user, body, and mode of governance are historical products of a scientific discourse that evolved around the IUD over fifty years under changing social circumstances.

Various discourses of difference helped rationalize the simultaneous existence of disparately positioned users. Blatantly discriminatory language was initially accepted for arguing that women who were considered incapable of contracepting autonomously should be given this imposable device. Such prejudiced language was later revised, and milder reasoning was used to rationalize unequal treatment. Economic feasibility, for example, became the rationale for not actively distributing Mirena in the global South and reinscribing the copper T as the satisfactory device for population management. Discrepancies in health care access legitimized childless women of the global South to be given the IUD in order to prevent health risks associated with pregnancy, while the same category of women in the global North were told that they should refrain from IUD use because it could jeopardize their future fertility.

While IUD developers emphasized differences among women to negotiate acceptable modes of governance for the device, they also assumed that women were biologically similar. Once biological similarities were foregrounded, differences among women were effaced, and a contraceptive technology was presumed to be universal. Research on the IUD standardized uterine physiology, quantified contraceptive performance, and used clinical trials to assess risks. These scientific activities erased physiological variations as well as sociocultural differences among prospective users and rendered the female body a measurable and controllable passive receptacle for the device. Privileging scientific explanations of fertilization and menstruation silenced women's subjective experiences of pregnancy and cultural meanings associated with bleeding. In addition to the scientific discourse that effortlessly converts diversely situated users into a homogenized female body, the rhetoric of choice is beginning to be applied globally without regard for inequities among women's positions. These discursive rearrangements have transformed a device that once targeted a specific group of women into a commonly applicable technology for all women.

In sum, the construction of a politically versatile technology entailed masking heterogeneous biopolitical scripts with a universalized technology. By obfuscating unequal global power relationships with the rhetoric of biological sameness, the scientific discourse has been able to depoliticize IUD development. In other words, constructing and obscuring differences among women, as well as concurrently appropriating and obliterating their agencies, were the two most important mechanisms that enabled diverse biopolitical agendas to become integral to this device.

The Technoscientific Body

This study also showed that implicated users were not merely rhetorical products. Discourse often shaped how women's bodies were understood and treated and how users experienced the IUD in real life. Constructed as the masses whose fertility needed to be brought under control, numerous women became targets of coercive and semicoercive insertions of IUDs. When developers envisioned the efficacy of the contraceptive method in terms of the device's sustained occupation of the uterus, this led to an unnecessary proliferation of infections and complications in IUD users around the world. When IUD providers put the rhetoric of the "safe" user into practice, women whose age, marital status, and sexual behavior made them risky were refused IUD insertions. The idea that less menstrual bleeding is an additional benefit shaped Mirena users' experiences; many found this side effect to be a liberating, unexpected bonus. The more expensive lifestyle technology was more easily withheld from women of the global South who were construed as not modern enough. Scientific discourse thus has had material, or real life, consequences.

Technoscience mediates the material realities of women's bodies in every corner of the world where contraceptives are distributed. Not only have female bodies been physically altered by technology, they have also been produced through material-semiotic practices of contraceptive discourses. The technoscientific body of an IUD user is an amalgamation of the heterogeneous constructions of bodies generated at various knowledge-power nexuses.

The Way Forward

Politically versatile technology such as the IUD defies the notion that technologies can be simply neutral, bad, or good. The examination of how political versatility was built into this product entailed the deconstruction of scientific knowledge claims as ideological constructs. Feminist theorists have long been critics of science, particularly in regard to how the pretense of objectivity and value neutrality masks masculinist biases in science. But for feminist activists who would have relied on science to light the path to morally higher grounds, the idea of science as a social construction may be problematic. At any rate, as chapter 4 in particular emphasized, we cannot rely on science alone to serve as the arbiter of inherently political issues. How, then, might feminists and feminist scholars confront the technoscientific body, its complex realities of global inequalities, and the simultaneous possibilities of empowerment and exploitation of women? I turn to the diffractive methodology to make a few proposals.

First, I believe that as we proceed, feminists must always feel conflicted. As diffractive patterns illuminated the network of meanings of the technoscientific body, they made apparent how technological interventions in diverse women's bodies are interconnected historically, transnationally, and theoretically. They also uncovered various forms of oppression involved in the making of a potentially beneficial technology. When we dissect the histories, the power relations, and the contradictions in meanings, we become cognizant of the conflicted relationships that our own technoscientific bodies rely on. This recognition should compel us to acknowledge the ironies and contradictions inherent in any particular feminist agenda, particularly ones we might support. Feeling ambivalent, I argue, is a state of feminist consciousness that is committed to a holistic vision.

Second, I suggest that feminist activists should not be afraid of pursuing the potentially empowering opportunities that a technological artifact could provide as long as we remain cautious about the possibility of exploitative aspects. Diffracting could uncover heterogeneous meanings associated with technoscience and help identify agendas we could advocate for without losing sight of potentially negative implications. Feminist scholars could apply the diffractive methodology to other topics and develop well-rounded critical perspectives that can assist in plotting progressive paths forward.

Finally, I believe that as a community, feminists must be willing to engage multiple agendas that empower diversely situated women. By making different patterns of life and history visible, diffractive methodology commands a political position that tolerates and incorporates heterogeneous significances and actions. This methodology also provides a tool to ascertain what meanings are operative in a specific time and place, thus enabling us to extend support for one another on various fronts without falling into relativism. Feminist scholars of color have already pointed out that the concept of reproductive rights is not relevant to the empowerment of women of color. But diffraction as a critical metaphor invites multiple feminist consciousnesses that move us beyond the notion that reproductive rights and reproductive justice are somehow exclusive concepts that apply to separate groups of women. Diffracted kaleidoscopic feminist visions should guide us to reformulate worn-out feminist methodologies and generate material-semiotic practices that enable new forms of feminist alliances to undo decades of violent occupation of our bodies.

Notes

Preface

1. Thanks to Barbara B. Crane for planting the seed in my mind that led to this book.

2. Takeshita (2010).

3. See Haraway (1988) and Harding (1991).

4. See Harris (2000).

5. Takeshita (2004).

Chapter 1

1. See Oudshoorn (2003b) for the history of the trajectories of male contraceptive development.

2. Clarke (2000, 50).

3. Whyte, van der Geest, and Hardon (2002, 13).

4. Foucault (1976). Biopower is discussed more fully later in this chapter.

5. Oudshoorn (1994) and Clarke (1998). Historical studies on the first female oral contraceptive also include Watkins (1998), Marks (2001), Briggs (2002), and Laveaga (2009).

6. Statistical ranking is according to the *World Contraceptive Use 2005* (United Nations, Department of Social and Economic Affairs) found at: http://www.un.org/esa/population/publications/contraceptive2005/WCU2005.htm. See D'Arcangues (2007) for information on the worldwide distribution of the IUD.

7. See Tandon (2010) for the story of Abi Santosh's attempt to eliminate the side effects of the copper T by coating the copper with biodegradable polymers in an effort to increase acceptance of this device. He is one of the sixty-seven researchers

selected for the Bill & Melinda Gates Foundation's award for innovations in global health improvement in 2010.

8. See McCullough (2010).

9. Seaman (1969).

10. Mintz (1985).

11. Seaman and Seaman (1977).

12. Grant (1992), Hicks (1994), and Hawkins (1997).

13. Tone (1999, 388).

14. Hartmann (1995).

15. Halfon (2007).

16. Dixon-Mueller (1993).

17. Feldt (2004).

18. Winner (1986) and MacKenzie and Wajcman (1999) represent these STS approaches. Haraway (1988) introduced the idea of situatedness.

19. Dugdale (1999, 2000).

20. Dugdale (1995). Her dissertation extends into the late 1980s, but the document is not easily accessible for the public.

21. Bashford (2008, 330).

22. See Connelly (2008) for a detailed historical account of the population establishment.

23. Ehrlich (1968).

24. See Barrett and Frank (1999) for prewar, interwar, and postwar transformations of the population problem as conceived in the international arena.

25. Barrett and Kurzman (2004).

26. Gordon (2007).

27. Ibid. (280).

28. Quoted in Grant (1992, 31) and Tone (1999, 380).

29. Davis (1971, 34).

30. Quoted in Connelly (2008, 166).

31. Connelly (2006, 220).

32. Connelly (2008, 166).

33. Ibid.

34. Connelly (2003, esp. 127).

35. Bashford (2007).

36. Bashford (2008).

37. Hodgson and Watkins (1997, esp. 472).

38. See note 2 in Barrett and Frank (1999, 318).

39. IUD models developed independent of the Population Council include the Saf-T-Coil, the Dalkon Shield, and the Copper-7, which were marketed independently by pharmaceutical companies and have since been withdrawn. A number of models developed in Europe are still in circulation, but not as widely as the devices developed by the council. China and other communist countries, such as the former Soviet Union, Cuba, and Vietnam, are large users of the device, whose efforts were independent of Western interventions. See Gu et al. (1994).

40. Population Council (1955, 5).

41. Onorato (1990).

42. Connelly (2008, 159).

43. Onorato (1990, 1567).

44. Ibid.

45. Connelly (2008).

46. Onorato (1990).

47. Ishihama (1959) and Oppenheimer (1959).

48. Population Council (1961, 19).

49. Onorato (1990, 162). The Population Council's preference for long-term imposable methods is noticeable in their choice of subdermal implant as its next major contraceptive development project after the IUD.

50. Onorato (1990, tables 7.4 and 7.5) provides details of the council's funding.

51. Population Council (1971, 1975, 1983).

52. Berelson (1965, 13).

53. Clarke and Montini (1993, 45) define "implicated actors" as those for whom actions taken "will be consequential, regardless of their current presence."

54. See the introduction of Oudshoorn and Pinch (2003) for an overview on STS approaches to users.

55. Oudshoorn (2000, 138).

56. van Kammen (2000).

57. Dugdale (2000).

58. Ibid. (167).

59. Woolgar (1991, 59).

60. Akrich (1992, 209).

61. Oudshoorn and Pinch (2003, 17). See also Lindsay (2003).

62. Oudshoorn and Pinch (2003).

63. Oudshoorn (2003a).

64. I elaborate on the notion of biopolitical script later in this chapter.

65. See Collins (2000) and Crenshaw (1991) for seminal work on intersectionality.

66. Haraway (1997). For an example of feminist scholarship employing diffraction to advocate change, see Clarke and Olsen (1999). Barad (2007) greatly expands on and employs diffractive methodology to develop the notion of agential realism through the examination of quantum mechanics.

67. Haraway (2000, 104).

68. Ibid. (81).

69. Ibid. (73).

70. Foucault (1976).

71. Foucault (1997, 242).

72. Sawicki (1991, 68).

73. Foucault (1976).

74. Foucault (1997).

75. Rabinow and Rose (2006, 200).

76. Connelly (2006).

77. Connelly (2008, 161).

78. See DiMoia (2008) and Kim (2008) for historical analyses of family planning programs in Taiwan and Korea.

79. See Greenhalgh (1994, 1995) and Greenhalgh and Li (1995).

80. Gammeltoft (1999).

81. See Connelly (2006, 2008). Barrett and Kurzman (2004) also portray the eugenics movement as global in scope.

82. Connelly (2006, 232).

83. Sawicki (1991).

84. Bartky (1988).

85. Ibid. (68).

86. McCann (2009).

87. Petchesky (1984).

88. *Prolife* is a linguistic turn of phrase employed by antiabortion campaigns that elides any reference to women's bodies at stake or pregnancy. It rhetorically reduces birth control to a desire to be "against life." Elsewhere in the book, I use the term *antichoice* instead of *prolife* to characterize their stance.

89. Sawicki (1991, 86).

90. Ibid. (83).

91. Clarke (1998, 205).

92. Greenhalgh (1994).

93. Stark (2000).

94. Krengel and Greifeld (2000).

95. Gammeltoft (1999).

96. Butler (2004, 187).

97. Rabinow and Rose (2006).

98. Patrick (2003).

99. This is not to suggest that biopower is insidiously oppressive. Even Foucault distanced himself from the idea that power over life is unambiguously nefarious. As Rabinow and Rose (2006) note, medicine, in particular, is a site "where one can observe the play of truth, power, and ethics in relation to the subject, and the possibility of a good life" (196).

100. The term *biopolitical subject* appears in Ong (1995). Ong focuses on the agency and resistance of immigrants (biopolitical subjects) who are subjected to medical co-optation. My emphasis is on the construction of the biopolitical subjects and the mechanisms behind it.

101. The first four conference proceedings were published as Tietze and Lewit (1962), Segal, Southam, and Shafer (1965), Hefnawi and Segal (1975), and Bardin and Mishell (1994). The proceedings of the fifth conference were published as a special edition of the journal *Contraception* 75 (6S) in 2007.

102. *Population Reports* were originally published through the George Washington University Medical Center's Department of Medical and Public Affairs under a contract with USAID. The journal moved to Johns Hopkins University in 1978. USAID supports the publication. Information on IUDs is published under series B of the *Population Reports*. They are: Orlans (1973), Huber et al. (1975), Piotrow, Rinehart, and Schmidt (1979), Liskin (1982), Treiman and Liskin (1988), and Salem (2006).

103. I had access to the Population Council Archives, Accessions I and II, at the Rockefeller Archive Center in New York, as well as the Planned Parenthood Archives at the Sophia Smith Archives in Northampton, Massachusetts.

104. Segal (2003).

105. See Mintz (1985), Grant (1992), Hicks (1994), and Hawkins (1997).

106. Dugdale (1995).

107. For the history of the fertility control movements, see Reed (1983), McCann (1994), Halfon (2000, 2007), and Gordon (2007). For the history of oral contraceptives, see Watkins (1998) and Marks (2001). For the history of Norplant, see Watkins (2010a, 2010b).

108. For an analysis of IUD users across geographical areas and different modes of empowerment and resistance, see Takeshita (2004).

Chapter 2

1. Tietze and Lewit (1962, 7).

2. Ibid.

3. Guttmacher (1969, 43).

4. Guttmacher's statement has been quoted by at least two feminist scholars and criticized as "gynecological Taylorism." See Grant (1992, 73) and Tone (1999, 384). Here, I offer a reading that links his description to a specific kind of power over the body.

5. Thanks to Adele Clarke for suggesting the term *technoscientific form of biopower.* Latour (1987) coined the term *technoscience* to indicate that science and technology are no longer distinctively separable and that the two domains develop in a co-constitutive manner. For more discussions on Michel Foucault's notion of biopower, see chapter 1.

6. See Comaroff (1993), Fausto-Sterling (1995), Carruthers (2003), and Mann (2003).

7. Merchant (1983) and Schiebinger (2004).

8. Fausto-Sterling (1995). Sarah Bartmann was a native southern African woman who was brought to Europe by the Dutch and exhibited in London and Paris for what was perceived to be unusual bodily features. "Hottentot" women like Bartmann

were believed to have elongated labia, which she never allowed curious scientists to observe while she was alive. Upon her death, French scientists who specialized in comparative anatomy seized the opportunity to scrutinize her body. Her skeleton and preserved brain and genitals were displayed in the Musée de l'Homme in Paris until 1974. Her remains were repatriated to her homeland in 2002.

9. See also Stoler (2008) and Adams and Pigg (2005).

10. Escobar (1998).

11. Greenhalgh (1996, 28).

12. Ibid. (27).

13. See Riedmann (1993) for this characterization based on her study of demographic surveys conducted in Nigeria, which found that Western assumptions about ideal reproduction patterns were imposed, while local views on fertility were devalued.

14. McCann (2009).

15. Ibid. (153).

16. Clarke (2000).

17. Oudshoorn (1994, 115).

18. McCann (1994, 13).

19. See Watkins (1998, 14).

20. For the social history of the pill, see Watkins (1998).

21. McCann (1994).

22. Gordon (2007, esp. 279). For earlier examples of co-optation of the birth control movement into the eugenics and family planning movements, see McCann (1994).

23. Gordon (2007, 286).

24. Oudshoorn (1994, 117).

25. Gordon (2007, 286).

26. Briggs (2002).

27. See Oudshoorn (1994, 125) and Ramirez de Arellano and Seipp (1983, 107).

28. Edris Rice-Wray cited in Oudshoorn (1994, 130).

29. The initial FDA approval in 1957 for the treatment of menstrual disorders allowed doctors to prescribe the drug for birth control off-label, or for an indication other than what the medication has been approved for by the FDA, until the drug was approved as the first hormonal contraceptive three years later.

30. See Tone (1999).

31. Ibid. (379).

32. Segal et al. (1965).

33. Ibid. (1).

34. Margulies (1962, 61).

35. Birnberg and Burnhill (1968, esp. 861).

36. Tietze quoted in Reed (1983, 307).

37. Tone (1999).

38. Dugdale (2000).

39. Alan F. Guttmacher to John G. Searle (December 1964) quoted in Watkins (1998, 70).

40. Tietze and Lewit (1962, 122).

41. Ibid.

42. A statement from Robert Willson in ibid. (124).

43. Population Council (1963, 13).

44. See also FDA (1968) for the twenty-eight inventors and devices listed in appendix 8, "List of Available Intrauterine Contraceptive Devices and Exhibits of Labeling Submitted by Some Manufactures."

45. See Hall (1962) and Tietze (1962).

46. Lippes (1962, 70).

47. "Better coverage" and "inadequate coverage" are from Davis and Israel (1965, 140, 141).

48. Burnhill and Birnberg (1965, 128).

49. Ibid. (130–131).

50. Kamal (1979).

51. Ibid. (24).

52. "Loose and lost" is from ibid. (26); "disoriented " and "cavity occupation" are from ibid. (24).

53. "Fit snugly" is from ibid. (17); "harmonious fit relationship" is from ibid. (16).

54. See "Foreword" in ibid. (17).

55. Ibid. (5–6).

56. Kapsalis (1997, 39).

57. See Carruthers (2003) and Mann (2003).

58. In terms of failure rate measured by accidental pregnancy, studies generally showed that the IUD compared favorably to other available methods: between 1 and 6 women out of 100 got pregnant in one year. However, when expulsions and removals were added in, too many women were abandoning the method, although the rate of closure varied from study to study. Reports range widely from 12 to 42 percent of users discontinuing the device in the first year. See Huber et al. (1975).

59. The term *reject* appears in Razzak (1962, 56), Mann (1962, 93), and Davis and Israel (1965, 40). "Escape" appears in Tietze (1962, 16) and Razzak (1962, 56). "Angry uterus" is in Kamal (1979, 28). "Sending a message" is in Davis (1971, 128).

60. "The uterus was ejectively responding" appears in Mann (1962, 91). "Habitual ejecters," "incompetent internal os," and "incapable" appear in Margulies (1962, 66).

61. "Uterine protest" and "in the form of cramps and bleeding" are from Davis (1971, 84). "In each case" is a statement by Margaret Jackson during the discussion session in the 1962 conference; see Tietze and Lewit (1962, 121). "Reacting violently" is in Wood (1971, 51). "Restless" is in Jackson (1962, 37).

62. Fausto-Sterling (1995, 361).

63. Davis and Israel (1965, 135).

64. See ibid. (138, figure 3): "Distribution graph of superior and inferior transfundal measurements in 25 normal, parous, premenopausal uteri."

65. Statement made by Howard Taylor, chair of the 1964 conference; see Segal, Southam, and Shafer (1965, 202).

66. Davis and Israel (1965, 140).

67. Ibid., 141.

68. See Davis (1971, 86, figure 31). The caption for this figure reads: "Disproportion between standard size linear intrauterine coils and loop devices and uterine cavity size results in a significant incidence of removals, principally for cramping and bleeding complications. The use of small, flexible devices has greatly reduced the incidence of patient complaints and medical removals."

69. Davis (1971, 151).

70. The author does not specify the race of the women from whom he obtained these sample uteruses. Universality of women's bodies is again assumed across race, ethnicity, and geographical areas even though skeletal body size differences may result in significant differences in the sizes of women's organs. Thanks to Jan Roselle for this insight.

71. Tone (1999, 374).

72. Davis (1971, 41–43).

73. Mintz (1985).

74. See ibid. and Grant (1992). The FDA put a moratorium on Dalkon Shield sales in December 1974. The company finally announced retrieval in August 1975.

75. Mintz (1985), Grant (1992), Hicks (1994), and Hawkins, (1997).

76. From "Statement of Maj. Russel J. Thomsen, M.D., Fort Polka La.," U.S. Congress, House, Subcommittee of the Committee on Government Operations, *Regulation of Medical Devices (Intrauterine Contraceptive Devices)*, 93d Cong., 1st sess. (Washington, DC: Government Printing Office, 1973). Reprinted in Tone (1997, 239–240).

77. Mintz (1985, 99).

78. Connelly (2008, 296).

79. Ibid. (297), emphasis mine.

80. Ibid. (219).

81. Ibid.

82. See Martin (1991) and Haraway (1991).

83. See Ruzek (1978). See also Mintz (1985), Grant (1992), Hicks (1994), and Hawkins (1997).

84. See Porter (1995, esp. 76–77). For other science and technology studies scholarship on quantification, see Porter (1992) and Callon and Muniesa (2005).

85. See Dugdale (1999).

86. See Tietze (1962). See also Tone (1999).

87. Weilerstein (1957).

88. Tietze and Lewit (1962, 7).

89. Ibid., (123).

90. Ibid. Dugdale (1995) documents the difficulties Christopher Tietze and Robert Dickenson encountered during the 1940s when they tried to publish a research paper on IUDs. This experience is in the background of Tietze's assertion that the medical community requires convincing.

91. Oudshoorn (1994).

92. Tietze and Lewit (1962, 136).

93. Tietze (1968).

94. Making adjustments for the behavior of contraceptive users in statistical analyses started in the 1930s with the invention of the Pearl Index, a simple technique to report the effectiveness of a contraceptive method in the form of number of unintended pregnancies over a total number of months or menstrual cycles of exposure by women in the clinical trial. See Oudshoorn (1994) and McCann (1994).

95. Meldrum (1996, 291).

96. Oudshoorn (1994).

97. Tietze (1969, 185).

98. Meldrum (1996, 291–292).

99. Oudshoorn (1994, esp. 132).

100. Tietze (1968).

101. Oudshoorn (1994, 136–137).

102. Dugdale (2000, 173).

103. Tone (1999, 384).

104. Statement made by E. Kessel in 1974, quoted in Huber et al. (1975, 39).

105. Wood (1970, 51).

106. Population Council (1966, 18).

107. Ibid. (16). See also Connelly (2008) for a story of John D. Rockefeller's meeting with President Ayub Khan of Pakistan in 1963. Khan explained that population program in Pakistan was ineffective due to lack of reliable contraceptives. When he was presented with a Lippes loop, Khan became extremely enthusiastic and announced that he would have every midwife in Pakistan inserting them within two weeks.

108. Population Council (1966, 19).

109. Ibid. (19).

110. See Connelly (2008, 214–231).

111. Ibid. (2008, 223).

112. "Panic" is from in Dandekar et al. (1976, 227).

113. Ibid. (194).

114. See Ahn (1974) and Freedman, Hermalin, and Sun (1973).

115. Dugdale (1995, esp. 211).

116. Population Council (1966).

117. Mahadevan et al. (1994).

118. International Planned Parenthood Federation (1974).

119. Planned Parenthood Federation of Korea (1973).

120. An intrauterine device known as the Ota ring, developed by a Japanese gynecologist in 1930, was widely tested in Taiwan and Korea. See Früstück (2003) and Kim (2008).

121. Connelly (2008).

122. DiMoia (2008).

123. Connelly (2008, 245).

124. Ibid.

125. Ibid.

126. Population Council (1973).

127. Ibid. (26).

128. Dugdale (1995).

129. See Greenhalgh (1994) and Gammeltoft (1999).

130. The Indonesian IUD insertion campaign is reported in Hartmann (1995).

131. Gammeltoft (1999).

132. Gutiérrez (2008, 40).

133. See Thompson (2000) and Ortega, Amuchstegui, and Rivas (1998).

134. Sanders (2000). The organization CRACK has since changed its name to Project Prevention.

135. Bland (2002).

136. Joyce (2003, 12). For more on the idea that artifacts have politics, see Winner (1986). For more on the idea that artifacts have agencies or that they are the nonhuman actants in a sociotechnical network, see Latour (1987, 1996) and Callon (1986).

137. Watkins (1998, 135).

Chapter 3

1. For a more detailed perspective on my academic and personal journey with an IUD, see Takeshita (2010).

2. In 2002, American physicians had not yet fully recovered from the impression that IUDs were a risky business. Stanwood et al. (2002), an American College of Obstetrics and Gynecology survey, found that 16 percent of the 400 respondents

believed that using the IUD in their practices puts them at risk of litigation; 20 percent of these respondents had not inserted an IUD in the past year. The survey also revealed that the number of prescriptions written for IUDs was an average of seven per year. Also in 2002, the *Pittsburgh Post-Gazette* published an article titled "Just Try Getting an IUD," a story about a woman who was faced with a reluctant doctor when she asked for an IUD. See Devoe (2002).

3. Mintz (1985).

4. See Mintz (1985), Perry and Dawson (1985), Bacigal (1990), Sobol (1991), Grant (1992), Hicks (1994), and Hawkins (1997).

5. For details, see Mintz (1985, esp. 53–66).

6. Tone (1999, 277–278).

7. Russel J. Thomsen, M.D., "A Basis for Food and Drug Administration and Federal Trade Commission Regulation of IUD Research, Production, and Promotion," testimony presented at the House Government Operations Committee Hearing, May 30, 1973. Population Council Archive, Accession II, AD 11.

8. Mintz (1973).

9. Christian (1974).

10. Ibid. (1974, 444). I discuss this 1967 questionnaire conducted by the FDA later in this chapter.

11. Culliton and Knopman (1974, 841).

12. Grant (1992, esp. 60).

13. See Mintz (1985).

14. See ibid.

15. Most claimants settled for $725 compensation in 1990. See Szaller (1999).

16. Forrest and Fordyce (1993).

17. Piccinino and Mosher (1998).

18. By the time Ortho Pharmaceuticals took the Lippes loop off the market in September 1985, it had faced about 200 lawsuits. Over the thirteen years that Searle had been manufacturing copper IUDs in the United States, about 800 lawsuits had been filed against the company on the grounds that the devices caused PID. Although the company won most of the suits, the legal fees associated with defending itself amounted to more than $1.5 million. Ortho ceased manufacturing and distributing the Lippes loop in September 1985, and in January 1986, Searle stopped distributing the Cu-7 and TCu200 in the United States. (although it continued to distribute them in other countries). See Ramirez and Starrs (1987).

19. The only IUD that remained available in the United States was Progestasert, a hormone-releasing IUD manufactured by Alza Corporation in California; it was supplied only to Planned Parenthood–affiliated clinics and physicians who had prescribed the product in the past. See Ramirez and Starrs (1987).

20. According to Forrest and Fordyce (1993), 96 percent of U.S. IUD users were satisfied with the method, topped only by those who used implants. We can certainly question the validity of this survey considering that the implants became a source of controversy soon after their introduction in the United States. Yet given that the copper IUDs were one of the few nonhormonal contraceptive options, it is possible that some women who do not tolerate hormonal methods well would have preferred the device as a birth control method.

21. See Clarke (1984).

22. See Forrest (1986).

23. See Ramirez and Starrs (1987).

24. See Schoen (2005).

25. Segal, Southam, and, Shafer (1965, 215).

26. See Schoen (2005).

27. Ibid. (67).

28. Ibid.

29. Schoen (2005) found that many women were given contraceptive services without any follow-up; thus, no information about their continued use or complications exists.

30. See García (1982). Anderson (2006) also found that physicians who led the American imperialist occupation of the Philippines in the early twentieth century and later became heads of urban public health departments in the United States brought neocolonial practices such as rigorous personal hygiene campaigns back with them to the inner-city immigrants and marginalized populations.

31. Tone (1999, esp. 382).

32. Westoff (1972).

33. The constructions of the "birth control for a nation" and the "birth control for the individual" are discussed in chapter 2. See also Alan Guttmacher's comments in Tietze and Lewit (1962, 7).

34. See Watkins (1998) for a detailed social history of oral contraceptives from 1950 to 1970.

35. See also Tone (1999).

36. See FDA (1968, appendix 8).

37. Not all dubious devices made it to the mass market: some were designed and patented but never manufactured; others were inserted in patients by inventor physicians but abandoned before they became a widely distributed product. The Lippes loop, Saf-T-Coil, Dalkon Shield, Copper-7, and Progestasert were the major models marketed to American physicians through medical journals. Ortho Pharmaceuticals introduced the Lippes loop in 1964. Julius Schmid Laboratories started selling the Saf-T-Coil in 1967. A. H. Robins began marketing the Dalkon Shield in 1971. G. D. Searle and Company entered the market with the Cu-7 in 1973 and the TCu 200 in 1978, which were differently shaped copper-bearing plastic devices. Alza Corporation introduced the Progestasert, a T-shaped hormone-releasing model in 1976. See Anonymous (1986).

38. Population Council Office, New York, NY, "SAF-T-COIL" RAC, memorandum, May 20, 1965, PC, Box 123, Folder 2257.

39. Saf-T-Coil advertisements found in *American Journal of Obstetrics and Gynecologists* (1969, 1971, 1974) and *Fertility and Sterility* (1971).

40. See Mintz (1985, esp. 69–88).

41. For more on earlier intrauterine contraception, see Wood (1971), Dugdale (1999), and Tone (2001).

42. Tietze and Lewit (1962, 8).

43. Conference participants for the most part seemed to agree with comments supporting the safety of intrauterine devices such as this one from Dr. Oppenheimer: "I myself have never seen any inflammation or infection as a result of wearing the ring" (Oppenheimer, 1962, 28), and this one from Dr. Hall: "Side effects are few and no serious complications were encountered" (Hall, 1962, 34). Trust in antibiotics is represented by comments such as: "Most of [the infections] appeared in the 1930's before sulfa drugs and antibiotics became available" (Tietze, 1962, 17), and, "In our antibiotic era, one of the main dangers of this method—pelvic infection—has become greatly reduced" (Lehfeldt, 1962, 47).

44. Dr. Oppenheimer stated in 1962: "I believe most of the pain is psychologically induced because people warned against the method until about two years ago" (Oppenheimer, 1962, 26). Dr. Jack Lippes complained, "These two patients could not be convinced that the devices had nothing to do with the discharge. I was again compelled, at the patients' requests, to remove two more rings" (Lippes, 1962, 73).

45. Jessen (1962, 44).

46. Tietze (1962, 18).

47. A statement made by Lazar Margulies at the 1964 international conference. Transcribed in Segal, Southam, and Shafer (1965, 206).

48. Scott (1968b, 41).

49. Ibid. (44).

50. The advisory committee's actions were limited to recommending sterile packaging and proper insertion techniques to minimize the risk of infection and perforation. The committee announced that "more serious adverse reactions associated with the IUD are rare" (FDA, 1968, 8). Although Roger Scott also published a short note of warning in *Obstetrics and Gynecology* (Scott, 1968a) and some other studies in the late 1960s showed signs of possibly serious problems associated with IUD use, the scientific community was generally slow to investigate the risks of IUDs.

51. See Watkins (1998) for details on the controversy over the safety of the pill that led to the inclusion of patient information inserts in oral contraceptives.

52. Jones, Beniger, and Westhoff (1980).

53. Watkins (1998, esp. 116).

54. Tone (1999, esp. 383).

55. When public concern about the safety of oral contraceptives was nearing its peak, Davis appeared on TV, inciting fears about the pill and announcing that some modern IUDs (including the Dalkon Shield) provided 99 percent protection. Davis attacked the pill, obviously hoping that IUDs would gain more popularity, while playing up "the notion that science and technology had come up with a 'modern' intrauterine device in a nick-of-time rescue" (Mintz, 1985, 38). One Washington reporter stated, "Dr. Hugh Davis, of Johns Hopkins University, testified that the possible side effects [of the pill] are so great, if the pill were a food product it would probably be ordered off the market" (Watkins, 1998, 111).

56. Ibid.

57. In August 1972, for instance, *Mademoiselle* ran an article on contraceptives that referred to the Dalkon Shield as the preferred modern method. See Mintz (1985).

58. Seaman (1969).

59. Boston Women's Health Collective (1973).

60. In his first year-end report, Gene Vadies, director of the college program at the Planned Parenthood World Population, reported being in contact with 299 colleges in the organization's effort to disseminate birth control information to college students and assist campuses in establishing birth control services. "College Program. Planned Parenthood World Population. Year End Report. July 1, 1971 to June 30, 1972." (Planned Parenthood Federation of America, New York, NY. Archive II, Box 55, Folder 86). The University of Hawaii, for example, reported distributing IUDs in 1970 and 1971 to, respectively, 3.4 percent and 11.9 percent of their campus family planning clinic patients. (Eleanore Nordyke and Charles Odom, "A Family Planning

Clinic on Campus: First Year Experience at the University of Hawaii," n.d., Planned Parenthood Federation of America, Archive II, Box 55, Folder 81.) A friend of mine also attests to obtaining her first Dalkon Shield at a New York campus clinic in 1972. Mintz (1985) also recounts the story of "Mary," who developed severe infections from a shield she obtained at the University of Colorado student health service in 1972.

61. Westoff (1972).

62. Mintz (1985, 106).

63. See Ruzek (1978). See also, Mintz 1985; Grant 1992; Hicks 1994; Hawkins (1997).

64. Zipper (1969).

65. Dugdale (1995, esp. 212).

66. Ibid. (211).

67. Orlans (1973).

68. Tietze and Lewit (1970).

69. Nathanson (1991). See also Dugdale (1995, esp. 215–216).

70. Dugdale (1995).

71. See Mintz (1985, esp. 104–105).

72. Rauh and Burket (1975, 244).

73. The company sold the Copper-7 and an early version of the copper T until 1986. Copper devices rapidly replaced inert plastic devices: by 1979, 80 percent of the U.S. sales consisted of copper-bearing devices. For details, see Liskin (1982).

74. Dugdale (1995, esp. 222).

75. Orlans (1973).

76. "Statement by Daniel R. Mishell, M.D., Sheldon J. Segal, Ph.D., and Christopher Tietze, M.D., for the Population Council before the Subcommittee on Intergovernmental Relations, House Committee on Government Operations," June 12, 1973, Population Council Archives, Accession II, AD 11.

77. See Tatum (1975, 1976).

78. Tatum et al. (1975).

79. Mishell (1975b).

80. See Clark (1975) and Mishell (1975a).

81. A. H. Robins rejected the wicking tail theory. The faulty tail theory was not accepted as official evidence in court. Judge Lord, who found A. H. Robins guilty,

however, believed that the tail accounted for the injuries. For examples of main-stream medical resources that support the wicking tail theory, see Canavan (1998) and Treiman et al. (1995).

82. Was the Dalkon Shield more dangerous than other IUDs? This question spurred various studies, reports, and debates over the subsequent twenty years. Studies on IUD-related deaths, pelvic inflammatory disease, and infertility were conducted, most of them reporting an increased risk with IUD use in general and significantly elevated risk for Dalkon Shield users. See, for example, Cates et al. (1976), Kaufman et al. (1983), Lee et al. (1983), and Lee, Rubin, and Borucki (1988). Some scientists, however, disagreed with the view that the shield was uniquely dangerous. See, for example, Kronmal, Whitney, and Mumford (1991) and Mumford and Kessel (1992). IUD supporters responded to these publications, disputing the claim that the shield was no different from other devices. See, for example, Burkman, et al. (1991) and Sivin (1993). Sivin, who is an affiliate of the Population Council, reviewed past stud-ies in his 1993 publication in which he meticulously singled out the Dalkon Shield as the major source of IUD-related injuries, infertility, and deaths. He also criticized reports written during the 1980s for failing to point out that the shield had inflated the rate of risk of infertility for all IUDs, making the contraceptive method appear more dangerous than it actually was. Emphasizing that copper-bearing IUDs had the lowest risk and the shield the highest, Sivin presented the copper T as physically dif-ferent from and superior to the previous generation of IUDs that had posed higher health risks.

83. Burkman (1981). The Women's Health Study was conducted between 1976 and 1978 with grants from the National Institute of Child Health and Human Develop-ment. It compared 1,447 women hospitalized with pelvic inflammatory disease to 3,453 controls.

84. Cramer et al. (1985).

85. Lee, Rubin, and Boruck (1988).

86. See Mintz (1985, esp. 194–195).

87. Ibid. (esp. 104–105).

88. Ibid. (esp. 105–106).

89. Ory (1978).

90. Anonymous (1985).

91. Dugdale (1995) details this lawsuit, which was particularly well orchestrated by the plaintiff lawyers, who had won an early Dalkon Shield product liability suit.

92. Treiman and Liskin (1988).

93. Sivin (1993).

94. WHO (1996).

95. Toulemon and Leridon (1998, 117).

96. Cramer et al. (1985, 947). Of the infertility clinic patients they studied, only 3 percent were women with more than two children. The rest either had none or only one.

97. See Treiman and Liskin (1988) and Klitsch (1988).

98. "The New IUD: Medical, Legal, and Social Issues: Highlights of a Symposium." Moderator: William J. Ledger, M.D., Somerville, N.J. : GynoPharma Inc. (VHS, 1988).

99. "One Contraceptive Can Fit Her Lifestyle to a 'T,'" advertisement of ParaGard T380A Intrauterine Copper Contraceptive, GynoPharma Inc. in *Obstetrics and Gynecology*, 77, no. 1 (1991).

100. Dugdale (1995, 242).

101. "The New IUD."

102. Watkins (1998).

103. The women's health movement during the 1960s and 1970s largely aimed to provide women information that would allow them to take charge of their own bodies and health. Women-authored self-help health books for women such as *Our Bodies, Ourselves* emerged during this time. See Boston Women's Health Collectives (1973).

104. Watkins (1998, 125).

105. Ibid. (134).

106. See Anonymous (2002).

107. For more discussion on embodying the IUD as its scholar, see Takeshita (2010).

108. Statement made in "The New IUD."

109. Changes observed between Treiman and Liskin (1988) and Treiman, et al. (1995).

110. Ramirez and Starrs (1987, 73).

111. Forrest (1986, 52).

112. Treiman and Liskin (1995).

113. Ramirez and Starrs (1987, 73), quoting *Networks, Family Health International*.

114. Ibid. (73), quoting the IPPF International Medical Advisory Panel.

115. See Dugdale (1995, esp. 241).

116. Ibid. (242) agrees with me on this speculation.

117. Van Kammen and Oudshoorn (2002).

118. Germain and Dixon-Muller (1993).

119. Ibid.

120. Ortho-McNeil Pharmaceuticals purchased the license to market ParaGard from GynoPharma in 1995 and then sold it to Duramed Pharmaceuticals in 2006.

121. Hubacher et al. (2001).

122. "Mirena is recommended for women who have had at least one child. This is because most of the medical research conducted on Mirena for FDA approval was among women who had at least one child. Only you and your healthcare provider can decide if Mirena is right for you." (http://www.mirena-us.com/faqs/index .jsp#70, accessed October 2010).

Chapter 4

1. J. C. Willke, "The IUD," http://www.lifeissues.org/abortifacients/IUD.html (accessed November 2010).

2. Tietze and Lewit (1962, 110).

3. Margulies (1962, 67).

4. Tietze (1962, 14).

5. Dr. Edris Rice-Wray also pointed out that the mechanism of action as it relates to abortion would be an issue in Mexico where she works. See Tietze and Lewit (1962, 135).

6. Public Health Services Leaflet No. 1066. U.S. Department of Health, Education and Welfare, 1963.

7. Segal, Southam, and Shafer (1965, 212).

8. Ibid. (213).

9. Ibid. (217).

10. *American Congress of Obstetrics and Gynecology Terminology Bulletin—Terms Used in Reference to the Fetus*, Chicago, A.C.O.G. September 1965.

11. J.C. Willke and Bradley Mattes, "Dispelling the myths behind conception, contraception and abortifacient drugs," February 2010, http://www.lifeissues.org/ abortifacients (accessed September 2007). Language has been revised on this Web site since I first retrieved this quotation. The message remains, however, that the IUD "causes early abortion."

12. For example, *Life Advocate* magazine reprinted "Word Wars" by Eugene Diamond, M.D., who writes: "The hidden agenda in ACOG's redefinition of `contraceptive' was to blur the distinction between agents preventing fertilization and those preventing implantation of the week-old embryo. Specifically, abortifacients such as IUDs, combination pills, minipills, progestin-only pills, injectables such as Pro-vera and, more recently, implantables such as Norplant, all are contraceptives by this definition" (http://www.lifeadvocate.org/mar_97/wars.html, accessed November 2010).

13. Davis (1971, 123).

14. Piotrow, Rinehart, and. Schmidt (1979).

15. I am drawing this conclusion by comparing the two *Population Reports,* B3 (1979) and B4 (1982). The descriptions of the IUD's mechanism of action in them are virtually the same, suggesting that no significant findings were made during this period. See Piotrow, Rinehart, and Schmidt (1979) and Liskin (1982).

16. See Petchesky (1984).

17. See Crane and Finkle (1989). In addition to the gag rule, the United States abruptly ceased funding to the United Nations Population Fund in 1986, accusing the organization of supporting the coercive population policy in China.

18. Segal (2003).

19. The memoir does not identify Willke by name, but Segal reiterated this story with vigor in our telephone conversation in June 2003, which he did without my prompting, leading me to believe that this particular encounter with Willke awakened his sense of urgency to defend against attacks on contraceptives by antichoice extremists.

20. Segal (2003, xxiv).

21. Ibid.

22. Segal et al. (1985).

23. Segal declined to affirm my speculation that subsequent research activities by him and his colleagues were politically motivated. He maintained that they were done in pursuit of scientific knowledge. E-mail communication, September 2003.

24. Wilcox et al. (1987), for instance, used a recent technology developed by Armstrong, Ehrlich, and Birkin (1984) to gain new insight.

25. Segal (2003, 100).

26. Segal, Rinehart, and Schmidt (1985). To be precise, Segal's study explained the reason a past study had found hCG in IUD users was that it mistook preovulation hCG surge as a sign of pregnancy.

27. Wilcox et al. (1987).

28. Ortiz and Croxatto (1987).

29. Sivin (1989).

30. Alvarez et al. (1988).

31. Several years later, Ortiz and Croxatto (2007) reevaluated Alvarez's eggs with an electronic microscope and concluded that two out of the fourteen eggs (14 percent) recovered from IUD users had been fertilized.

32. *Webster* v. *Reproductive Health Services,* 492 U.S. 490 (1989). The full text can be found at http://www.law.cornell.edu/supct/html/historics/USSC_CR_0492_0490 _ZX.html (accessed November 2010).

33. Sivin (1989, 355).

34. Mason (2002, 226, note 40).

35. Ibid. (142). Antiabortion extremists also use the term *contraceptive mentality* to condemn what they see as the manipulation of production of human life in opposition to God's will.

36. Petchesky (1984, 264).

37. Mason (2002).

38. Petchesky (1984, 25).

39. J. C. Willke, "The IUD," http://www.lifeissues.org/abortifacients/IUD.html (accessed November 2010).

40. Ibid.

41. Ibid.

42. Spinnato (1997).

43. Ibid. (503).

44. Ibid. (505). For example, he dismisses Frank Alvarez's 1988 microscopic studies of eggs, maintaining that the timing of egg recovery was uncontrolled, numbers of subjects were too small, and 36 percent of the ova retrieved from IUD users had degenerated too much to determine whether they had ever been fertilized.

45. Segal (1997, 980).

46. Larimore (1999). Canavan (1998).

47. Canavan (1999).

48. See The American Academy of Family Physicians, "The Intrauterine Device (IUD)," December 1998, http://www.aafp.org/afp/981200ap/981200c.html (accessed November 2010). The exact language on the handout is: "The IUD prevents sperm

from joining with an egg. It does this by making the sperm unable to go into the egg and by changing the lining of the uterus."

49. See Fan and Zheng (1997). The range cited here is extrapolated from Koh and Jones (1982), which resulted in a 25 percent false-positive EPF diagnosis, or embryonic loss after fertilization was detected; Smart et al. (1983), which yielded 36 percent early pregnancy loss around implantation; Rolfe (1982), which found 78 percent loss within the first fourteen days; and Fan and Zheng (1997), which concluded that they observed false-positive early pregnancy tests at a rate of 17 percent. In Fan and Zheng's study, thirty-five of seventy women who were trying to conceive showed positive EPF two to seven days after ovulation. Twenty-eight of the thirty-five were confirmed to be pregnant during "follow-up," the timing and method of which are unspecified. There were seven cases of false positives and one case of a false negative.

50. Kennedy (1997, 729).

51. Wilcox, Baird, and Weinberg (1999).

52. Sivin (1989, 358).

53. Stanford and Mikolajczyk (2002).

54. Ibid. (1705).

55. Ibid.

56. Spinnato (1997, 503).

57. Larimore (1989, 761).

58. See Martin (1991) for how the medicalization of reproduction has affected women's perception of menstruation, pregnancy, childbirth, and menopause.

59. Brodie (1994).

60. In the future, earlier pregnancy detection methods available over the counter may enable women to find out within a few days that fertilization has occurred. Current early pregnancy factor detection methods that look for an indication that fertilization has occurred require a blood test and are available only clinically.

61. De Irala et al. (2007).

62. Porter (1995, ix).

63. For discussions on governing at a distance, see Rose and Miller (1992).

64. Spinnato (1997, 505).

65. Ibid..

66. Ibid..

67. Ibid..

68. McCann (1994, 18).

69. Ibid..

70. Hodgson and Watkins (1997, 480).

71. See chapters 1 and 2.

72. Population Council (1966, 19). Also quoted in Bruce (1987, 360).

73. See Matthew (2008, 297).

74. Population Council (1976, 20).

75. Bruce (1990).

76. Bruce (1987).

77. See Hodgson and Watkins (1997); Connelly, (2008).

78. Sen, Germain, and Chen (1994).

79. United Nations (1995).

80. Hartmann (1995).

81. For detailed discussion on how "women's empowerment" and "unmet need" have been appropriated in the post-Cairo population network, see Halfon (2000, 2007).

82. For instance, the Population Council's Reproductive Health Program aims to increase access to family planning and other reproductive health services in countries with unmet need. See http://www.popcouncil.org/what/rh.asp (accessed November 2010). UNFPA raises "failure to offer a wide selection of methods" and not being able to fulfill the "unmet need" as reasons that contraceptive services are not being utilized by women in developing countries: http://www.unfpa.org/rh/planning.htm (accessed November 2010).

83. Haberland and Measham (2002).

84. Connelly (2008).

85. Hartmann (1995).

86. Hodgson and Watkins (1997).

87. Halfon (2007).

88. The earliest reference to the cafeteria offering that I have found is in the conference proceedings of the 1964 international meeting on the IUD, when participants conceded that both the pill and the IUD should be in the mix of methods offered to women in the global South in order to ensure better compliance. See "Summation" by Alan F. Guttmacher in Segal Southam, and Shafer (1965, 217).

89. Oudshoorn (1996).

90. As noted above, IUD supporters were using the term *cafeteria* as early as 1964, which dates further back than Oudshoorn's explanation that the capitalist framework validated the cafeteria approach.

91. For more discussions on reconstructing the IUD as contraceptive choice, see Takeshita (2004).

92. Feldt (2004, 200).

93. It is important to note that other feminist scholars have expressed concerns over IUD abuse against underprivileged Mexican women, particularly of indigenous origin. See Ortega, Amuchstegui, and Rivas (1998) and Thompson (2000).

94. See Smith (2005).

95. Ibid. (133).

96. Ibid. (130).

97. Segal (2003, 205).

98. Ibid.

99. See Stangel (2009).

100. Latour (2003).

101. Mooney (2005).

102. Segal, Southam, and Shafer (1985).

103. Wilcox et al. (1987).

104. Alvarez et al. (1988).

105. It appears that funding to conduct further studies is also difficult to come by. I made this observation during the Q&A session at the fifth international conference on the IUD in 2005. Horacio Croxatto, in response to a question from the audience, stated that scarce funds were partly responsible for the lack of new findings on the mechanism of action of the hormone-releasing device.

Chapter 5

1. For more detailed perspective on my academic and personal journey with an IUD, see Takeshita (2010).

2. Posting on an online medication discussion resource, medications.com: http://www.medications.com/effect/view/34880 (accessed November 2010).

3. See for example, http://lifeaftermirena.blogspot.com

4. See Mamo and Fosket (2009).

5. See Loe (2004) and Mamo and Fishman (2004).

6. Blum and Stracuzzi (2004).

7. Scommegna et al. (1970).

8. Ibid. (201, 202).

9. Ibid. (209).

10. See Scommegna et al. (1974). This research was also funded by the Ford Foundation. This time, they tested a T-shaped progesterone-releasing device in 249 women for twelve months. No pregnancies resulted.

11. See Huber et al. (1975) and Piotrow, Rinehart, and Schmidt (1979).

12. See Segal (2003).

13. Population Council (1970).

14. Norplant consists of six levonorgestrel-containing matchstick-size rods that are implanted beneath the skin of a woman's forearm to prevent pregnancy for five years.

15. Prager and Darney (2007).

16. Moskowitz, Jennings, and Callahan (1995, S1).

17. See Watkins (2010a, 2010b).

18. Smith (2005b).

19. Moskowitz, Jennings, and Callahan (1995, S2).

20. The documentary film *Skin Deep* by Frances Reid records testimonies of women who suffered side effects from Norplant. See Reid (1995).

21. This report, Moskowitz, Jennings, and Callahan (1995), from the Hastings Center has been published as an edited volume: Moskowitz and Jennings (1996).

22. Huber et al. (1975, B-38).

23. "Uterine tranquilizer" appears in ibid.

24. See Tietze and Lewitt (1968).

25. See Liskin (1982).

26. See Treiman and Liskin (1988).

27. See Bernard (1970).

28. Whelan (1975).

29. Piotrow, Rinehart, and Schmidt (1979, B-66).

30. The WHO (1981) study was conducted between 1973 and 1979 and involved 5,322 parous women from fourteen cultural groups in Egypt, India (Hindu high caste, Hindu low caste), Indonesia (Javanese, Sudanese), Jamaica, Korea, Mexico, Pakistan (Punjab, Sind), the Philippines, United Kingdom, and Yugoslavia (Muslim, non-Muslim).

31. See Liskin (1982).

32. WHO (1981, 12).

33. See Liskin (1982).

34. WHO (1981, 13).

35. Chatterjee and Riley (2001).

36. The continuation rates for the levonorgestrel IUD were 74.5, 58.7, and 38.8 percent at one, two, and three years respectively. The continuation of copper devices ranged from 82.4 to 84.4 percent at year 1, 66.6 to 69.9 percent at year 2, and 45.4 to 50.4 percent at year 3. This was a double-blind trial, which disallowed physicians to provide consultation to women who received the LNG-IUD about possible amenorrhea. Thus the high discontinuation rate may have partly been corrected with counseling. See Indian Council of Medical Research (1989).

37. See Sivin et al. (1991).

38. Treiman et al. (1995).

39. Ibid. For the original report of the European study, see Andersson, Odlind, Goran Ryobo (1994).

40. Luukkainen (1994).

41. Ibid. (39).

42. Martin (2001).

43. See Pigg (2001). See also Adams and Pigg (2005).

44. Jim Shelton, "IUD Mirena," Dr. Jim Shelton's Pearls. January 15, 2001. http://info.k4health.org/pearls/2001/01-15.shtml (accessed November 2010) Shelton explains: "In the private sector at least, the price is likely to be in the hundreds of dollars. Over the years AID staff have had discussions with Schering (and with its predecessor Leiras) about an acceptable public sector price. Although we have never been able to reach accord, we will keep trying." USAID was not supplying Mirena at the time of writing this book.

45. Under their agreement, product donations to international development agencies and public health organizations can be made up to 1 percent of non-U.S. market

unit sales (about 53,000 IUDs by 2007). In addition, the company will sell up to 3 percent of non-U.S. market unit sales for under $40 to qualified public sector organizations. ICA has projects in Brazil, Curaçao, Dominican Republic, Ecuador, El Salvador, Ghana, Kenya, Indonesia, Nigeria, Paraguay, Saint Lucia, and South Africa. http://www.ica-foundation.org/ (accessed November 2010).

46. Rademacher et al. (2009). Available at http://www.k4health.org/toolkits/iud/essential-knowledge-about-lng-ius (accessed November 2010).

47. These cost figures are based on my own experience between 2002 and 2005. Prices vary depending on the provider, and distributors' business decisions may affect future prices.

48. ARCH Foundation, http://www.archfoundation.com/ (accessed November 2010).

49. Rademacher et al. (2009). See also Trussell, Lalla, and Doan (2008).

50. Faundesa et al. (1988).

51. Luukkainen and Toivonen (1995).

52. Ibid. (274).

53. See Fraser (2007).

54. See Rarick (2007).

55. Oudshoorn (1994, 121).

56. Ibid.

57. Coutinho and Segal (1999, 163).

58. Ibid.

59. Ibid. (164).

60. Ibid.

61. Mamo and Fosket (2009, 933).

62. Ibid. (931).

63. Mirena promotional material from October 2006 for prescribing physicians.

64. See note 2.

65. Joyce (2003, 4).

66. Kapsalis (1997).

67. Ibid. (53).

68. ParaGard product Web site: http://www.paragard.com/home.php (accessed November 2010).

69. Mirena product Web site: http://www.mirena-us.com/index.jsp (accessed November 2010).

70. Collins (1999, 266).

71. www.ica-foundation.org (accessed November 2010).

Chapter 6

1. Haraway (1997, 218, 273).

References

Archival Materials

Planned Parenthood Federation of America Papers, Sophia Smith Collection, Smith College, Northampton, MA.

Population Council Papers, Rockefeller Archives Center, Tarrytown, NY.

Published Sources

Adams, Vincanne, and Stacy Leigh Pigg. 2005. *Sex in Development: Science, Sexuality, and Morality in Global Perspective*. Durham, NC: Duke University Press.

Ahn, S. K. 1974. "The Korean National Family Planning Program." In *Population and Family Planning in the Republic of Korea*. Seoul, Korea: Korean Institute for Family Planning.

Akrich, Madeleine. 1992. The De-Scription of Technical Objects. In *Shaping Technology/Building Society*. Edited by Weibe Bijker and John Law. Cambridge, MA: MIT Press.

Alvarez, F. V., V. Brache, E. Fernandez, B. Guerrero, E. Guiloff, and R. Hess. 1988. New Insights on the Mode of Action of Intrauterine Contraceptive Devices in Women. *Fertility and Sterility* 49:768–773.

Anderson, Warwick. 2006. *Colonial Pathologies: Hygiene, Race, and Science in the Philippines*. Durham, NC: Duke University Press.

Andersson, Kerstin, Viveca Odlind, and Goran Ryobo. 1994. Levonorgestrel-Releasing and Copper-Releasing (Nova T) IUDs during Five Years of Use: A Randomized Comparative Trial. *Contraception* 49:56–71.

Anonymous. 1985. Ortho Stops Marketing Lippes Loop; Cites Economic Factors. *Contraceptive Technology Update* 6 (11): 149–152.

Anonymous. 1986. G. D. Searle Withdraws Copper IUD, Leaving Only One, Little-Used Device on U.S. Market. *Family Planning Perspectives* 18 (1): 35.

Anonymous. 1988. *The New IUD: Medical, Legal, and Social Issues—Highlights from a Symposium.* Somerville, N.J.: GynoPharma Inc. (VHS)

Anonymous. 2002. Trial Court Properly Dismissed IUD Suit Because User Knew the Risks. *Medical Devices Litigation Reporter* 9 (6): 12.

Armstrong, E. G., P. H. Ehrlich, and S. Birkin. 1984. Use of a Highly Sensitive and Specific Immunoradiometric Assay for Detection of Human Chorionic Gonadotropin in Urine of Normal, Nonpregnant, and Pregnant Individuals. *Journal of Clinical Endocrinology and Metabolism* 59:867–874.

Bacigal, Ronald J. 1990. *Limits of Litigation: The Dalkon Shield Controversy.* Durham, NC: Carolina Academic Press.

Barad, Karen. 2007. *Meeting the Universe Halfway: Quantum Physics and the Entanglement of Matter and Meaning.* Durham, NC: Duke University Press.

Bardin, Wayne C., and Daniel R. Mishell, eds. 1994. *Proceedings from the Fourth International Conference on IUDs.* Newton, MA: Butterworth-Heinemann.

Barrett, Deborah, and David John Frank. 1999. Population Control for National Development: From World Discourse to National Policies. In *Constructing World Culture: International Nongovernmental Organizations since 1875.* Edited by John Boli and George M. Thomas. Palo Alto, CA: Stanford University Press.

Barrett, Deborah, and Charles Kurzman. 2004. Globalizing Social Movement Theory: The Case of Eugenics. *Theory and Society* 33 (5): 487–527.

Bartky, Sandra. 1988. Foucault, Femininity and the Modernization of Patriarchal Power. In *Feminism and Foucault: Reflections on Resistance.* Edited by Lee Quinby and Irene Diamond. Boston: Northeastern University Press.

Bashford, Alison. 2007. Nation, Empire, Globe: The Spaces of Population Debate in the Interwar Years. *Comparative Studies in Society and History* 49 (1): 170–201.

Bashford, Alison. 2008. Population, Geopolitics, and International Organizations in the Mid Twentieth Century. *Journal of World History* 19 (3): 327–348.

Berelson, Bernard. 1965. Application of Intra-Uterine Contraception in Family Planning Programs. In *Intra-Uterine Contraception: Proceeding of the Second International Conference, October 2–3, 1964, New York City.* Edited by Sheldon Segal, Anne Southam, and K. D. Shafer. New York: Excerpta Medica Foundation.

Bernard, R. R. 1970. IUD Performance Patterns: A 1970 World View. *International Journal of Gynaecology and Obstetrics* 8 (6): 926–940.

Birnberg, Charles H., and Michael Burnhill. 1968. Whither the IUD? The Present and Future of Intrauterine Contraceptives. *Obstetrics and Gynecology* 31:861.

Bland, Karina. 2002. Addicts Get Cash for Birth Control. Associated Press Newswire, July 28.

Blum, Linda M., and Nena Stracuzi. 2004. Gender in the Prozac Nation: Popular Discourse and Productive Femininity. *Gender and Society* 18 (3): 269–286.

Boston Women's Health Collective. 1973. *Our Bodies, Ourselves*. New York: Simon and Schuster.

Briggs, Laura. 2002. *Reproducing Empire: Race, Sex, Science, and U.S. Imperialism in Puerto Rico*. Berkeley: University of California Press.

Brodie, Janet Farrell. 1994. *Contraception and Abortion in the Nineteenth Century*. Ithaca, NY: Cornell University Press.

Bruce, Judith. 1987. Users' Perspectives on Contraceptive Technology and Delivery Systems: Highlighting Some Feminist Issues. *Technology in Society* 9 (3–4): 359–383.

Bruce, Judith. 1990. Fundamental Elements of the Quality of Care: A Simple Framework. *Studies in Family Planning* 21 (2): 61–91.

Burkman, Ronald T. 1981. Association between the Intrauterine Device and Pelvic Inflammatory Disease. *Obstetrics and Gynecology* 57:269–276.

Burkman, Ronald T., Nancy C. Lee, Howard W. Ory, and George L. Rubin. 1991. Response to the Intrauterine Device and Pelvic Inflammatory Disease: The Women's Health Study Reanalyzed. *Journal of Clinical Epidemiology* 44:123–125.

Burnhill, Michael, and Charles H. Birnberg. 1965. Superimposition Hysterography as a Tool in the Investigation of Intra-Uterine Contraceptive Devices: Preliminary Report. In *Intra-Uterine Contraception: Proceedings of the Second International Conference, October 2-3, 1964, New York City, Sponsored by the Population Council*, edited by S. J. Segal, A. L. Southam, and K.D. Shafer. New York: Excerpta Medica. 127–134.

Butler, Judith. 2004. Bodies and Power Revisited. In *Feminism and the Final Foucault*. Edited by Dianna Taylor and Karen Vintges. Urbana: University of Illinois Press.

Callon, Michel. 1986. Some Elements of a Sociology of Translation: Domestication of the Scallops and the Fishermen of St. Brieuc Bay. In *Power, Action and Belief: A New Sociology of Knowledge*. Edited by John Law. London: Routledge & Kegan Paul.

Callon, Michel, and Fabian Muniesa. 2005. Markets as Calculative Collection Devices. *Organization Studies* 26 (8): 1229–1250.

Canavan, Timothy P. 1998. Appropriate Use of the Intrauterine Device. *American Family Physician* 58 (9): 2077–2088.

Canavan, Timothy P. 1999. The Potential Postfertilization Effect with Use of the IUD. In Reply. *American Family Physician* 60 (3): 761.

Carruthers, Jane. 2003. Friedrich Jeppe: Mapping the Transvaal c.1850–1899. *Journal of Southern African Studies* 29 (4): 955–976.

Cates, Willard, Jr., Howard W. Ory, Roger W. Rochat, and Carl W. Tyler Jr.. 1976. The Intrauterine Device and Deaths from Spontaneous Abortion. *New England Journal of Medicine* 295 (21): 1155–1159.

Chatterjee, Nilanjana, and Nancy E. Riley. 2001. Planning an Indian Modernity: The Gendered Politics of Fertility Control. *Signs: Journal of Women in Culture and Society* 26 (31): 811–845.

Christian, C Donald. 1974. Maternal Deaths Associated with an Intrauterine Device. *American Journal of Obstetrics and Gynecology* 119:441–444.

Clark, Frederick A. 1975. The IUD Revisited. *Family Planning Perspectives* 7 (6): 245–246.

Clarke, Adele. E. 1984. Subtle Sterilization Abuse: A Reproductive Rights Perspective. In *Test Tube Women: What Future for Motherhood?* Edited by R. Arditti, R. D. Klein, and S. Minden. Boston: Pandora/Routledge and Kegan Paul.

Clarke, Adele E. 1998. *Disciplining Reproduction: Modernity, American Life Sciences, and "the Problem of Sex."* Berkeley: University of California Press.

Clarke, Adele E. 2000. Maverick Reproductive Scientists and the Production of Contraceptives, 1915–2000+. In *Bodies of Technology: Women's Involvement with Reproductive Medicine*. Edited by A. R. Saetnan, Nelly Oudshoorn, and M. Kirejczyk. Columbus: Ohio State University.

Clarke, Adele. 2008. Introduction: Gender and Reproductive Technologies in East Asia. *EASTS: East Asian Science and Technology Studies: An International Journal* 2 (3): 303–326.

Clarke, Adele E., and Theresa Montini. 1993. The Many Faces of Ru486: Tales of Situated Knowledges and Technological Contestations. *Science, Technology and Human Values* 18 (1): 42–77.

Clarke, Adele. E., and Virginia L. Olsen. 1999. *Revisioning Women, Health, and Healing: Feminist, Cultural, and Technoscience Perspectives*. New York: Routledge.

Collins, Patricia Hill. 2000. *Black Feminist Thought: Knowledge, Consciousness and the Politics of Empowerment*. New York: Routledge.

Collins, Patricia Hill. 1999. Will the "Real" Mother Please Stand Up? The Logic of Eugenics and American National Family Planning. In *Revisioning Women, Health, and Healing: Feminist, Cultural, and Technoscience Perspectives*. Edited by Adele. E. Clarke and Virginia L. Olsen. New York: Routledge.

Comaroff, Jean. 1993. The Diseased Heart of Africa: Medicine, Colonialism, and the Black Body. In *Knowledge, Power and Practice: The Anthropology of Medicine and Everyday Life*. Edited by Shirley Lindenbaum and Margaret Locks. Berkeley: University of California Press.

Connelly, Matthew. 2003. Population Control Is History: New Perspectives on International Campaign to Limit Population Growth. *Comparative Studies in Society and History* 45 (1): 122–147.

Connelly, Matthew. 2006. Seeing Beyond the State: The Population Control Movement and the Problem of Sovereignty. *Past and Present* 193 (1): 197–233.

Connelly, Matthew. 2008. *Fatal Misconception: The Struggle to Control World Population.* Cambridge, MA: Harvard University Press.

Coutinho, Elsimar, and Sheldon J. Segal. 1999. *Is Menstruation Obsolete?* New York: Oxford University Press.

Cramer, Daniel W., Isaac Schiff, Stephen C. Schoenbaum, Mark Gibson, Serge Belisles, Bruce Albrecht, Robert J., Stillman, Merle J. Berger, Emery Wilson, Bruce V. Stadel, and Machelle Seibel. 1985. Tubal Infertility and the Intrauterine Device. *New England Journal of Medicine* 312 (15): 941–947.

Crane, Barbara B., and Jason L. Finkle. 1989. The United States, China, and the United Nations Population Fund: Dynamics of U.S. Policy Making. *Population and Development Review* 15 (1): 23–59.

Crenshaw, Kimberle. 1991. Mapping the Margins: Intersectionality, Identity Politics, and Violence against Women of Color. *Stanford Law Review* 43 (6): 1241–1299.

Culliton, Barbara, and Debra S. Knopman. 1974. Dalkon Shield Affair: A Bad Lesson in Science and Decision Making. *Science* 185:839–841.

D'Arcangues, Catherine. 2007. Worldwide Use of Intrauterine Devices for Contraception. *Contraception* 75:S2–S7.

Dandekar, Kumudini, Vaijayanti Bhate, Jeroo Coyaji, and Surekha Nikam. 1976. Place of IUD in the Contraception-Kit of India. *Artha Vijnana* 18 (3): 189–286.

Davis, Hugh J. 1971. *Intrauterine Devices for Contraception: The IUD.* Baltimore, MD: Williams & Wilkins.

Davis, Hugh J., and R. Israel. 1964. Uterine Cavity Measurements in Relation to Design of Intra-Uterine Contraceptive Devices. In *Intra-Uterine Contraception: Proceedings of the Second International Conference, October 2–3, 1964, New York City, Sponsored by the Population Council.* Edited by S. J. Segal, A. L. Southam, and K. D. Shafer. New York: Excerpta Medica.

de Irala, J., C. L. del Burgo, C. M. L. de Fez, J. Arredondo, R. T. Mikolajczyk, and J. B. Stanford. 2007. Women's Attitudes towards Mechanism of Action of Family Planning Methods: Survey in Primary Health Centres in Pamplona, Spain. *BMC Women's Health* 7:10–19.

Devoe, Jan. 2002. Clearing Up Misconceptions about IUDs. *Pittsburgh Post-Gazette,* April 9, E-4.

DiMoia, John. 2008. Let's Have the Proper Number of Children and Raise Them Well: Family Planning and Nation-Building in South Korea, 1961–1968. *EASTS: East Asian Science and Technology Studies: An International Journal* 2 (3): 361–379.

Dixon-Mueller, Ruth. 1993. *Population Policy and Women's Rights: Transforming Reproductive Choice*. Westport, CT: Praeger.

Dugdale, Anni. 1995. *Devices and Desires: Constructing the Intrauterine Device, 1908–1988*. Science and Technology Studies, PhD diss., University of Wollongong.

Dugdale, Anni. 1999. Inserting Grafenberg's IUD into the Sex Reform Movement. In *The Social Shaping of Technology*. 2nd ed. Edited by Donald MacKenzie and Judy Wajcman. Buckingham: Open University Press.

Dugdale, Anni. 2000. Intrauterine Contraceptive Devices, Situated Knowledges, and Making of Women's Bodies. *Australian Feminist Studies* 15 (32): 165–176.

Ehrlich, Paul R. 1968. *The Population Bomb*. Cutchogue, NY: Buccaneer Books.

Escobar, Arturo. 1998. *Encountering Development: The Making and Unmaking of the Third World*. Princeton, NJ: Princeton University Press.

Fan, Xiao-Guang, and Zhen-Qun Zheng. 1997. A Study of Early Pregnancy Factor Activity in Preimplantation. *American Journal of Reproductive Immunology* 37:359–364.

Faundesa, Anibal, Francisco Alvarez, V. Bracheb, and A. S. Tejadab. 1988. The Role of the Levonorgestrel Intrauterine Device in the Prevention and Treatment of Iron Deficiency Anemia during Fertility Regulation. *International Journal of Gynaecology and Obstetrics* 26:429–433.

Fausto-Sterling, Anne. 1995. Gender, Race, and Nation: The Comparative Anatomy of Hottentot Women in Europe, 1815–1817. In *Deviant Bodies: Critical Perspectives on Difference in Science and Popular Culture*. Edited by Jennifer Terry and Jacqueline Urla. Bloomington: Indiana University Press.

FDA. 1968. *Report on Intrauterine Contraceptive Devices*. Edited by Advisory Committee on Obstetrics and Gynecology. Washington, DC: Food and Drug Administration.

Feldt, Gloria. 2004. *The War on Choice: The Right-Wing Attack on Women's Rights and How to Fight Back*. New York: Bantam Books.

Forrest, Jacqueline D. 1986. The End of IUD Marketing in the United States: What Does It Mean for American Women? *Family Planning Perspectives* 18:52–57.

Forrest, Jacqueline D., and R. R. Fordyce. 1993. Women's Contraceptive Attitudes and Use in 1992. *Family Planning Perspectives* 25 (4): 175–179.

Foucault, Michel. 1976. *History of Sexuality: Introduction*. New York: Vintage Books.

Foucault, Michel. 1997. *Society Must Be Defended, Lectures at the College De France, 1975-1976.* New York: Picador.

Fraser, Ian. 2007. The Promise and Reality of the Intrauterine Route for Hormone Delivery for Prevention and Therapy of Gynecological Disease. *Contraception* 75 (S6): S112–S117.

Freedman, R., A. I. Hermalin, and T. H. Sun. 1973. Fertility Trends in Taiwan: 1961–1970. In *Essays on the Population of Taiwan.* Edited by P. K. C. Liu. Taipei, Taiwan: Academia Sinica.

Frustuck, Sabine. 2003. *Colonizing Sex: Sexology and Social Control in Modern Japan.* Berkeley: University of California Press.

Gammeltoft, Tine. 1999. *Women's Bodies, Women's Worries: Health and Family Planning in a Vietnamese Rural Community.* Surrey: Curzon Press.

García, Ana Maria. 1982. *La Operación.* New York: Cinema Guild (VHS).

Germain, Adrienne, and Ruth Dixon-Muller. 1993. Whose Life Is It, Anyway? Assessing the Relative Risks of Contraception and Pregnancy. In *Four Essays on Birth Control Needs and Risks.* Edited by Ruth Dixon-Muller and Adrienne Germain. New York: International Women's Health Coalition.

Gordon, Linda. 2007. *The Moral Property of Women: A History of Birth Control Politics in America.* Chicago: University of Illinois Press.

Grant, Nicole J. 1992. *The Selling of Contraception: The Dalkon Shield Case, Sexuality, and Women's Autonomy.* Columbus: Ohio State University Press.

Greenhalgh, Susan. 1994. Controlling Births and Bodies in Village China. *American Ethnologist* 21 (1): 3–30.

Greenhalgh, Susan, ed. 1995. *Situating Fertility: Anthropology and Demographic Inquiry.* Cambridge: Cambridge University Press.

Greenhalgh, Susan. 1996. The Social Construction of Population Science: An Intellectual, Institutional, and Political History of Twentieth-Century Demography. *Comparative Studies in Society and History* 38 (1): 26–66.

Greenhalgh, Susan, and Jiali Li. 1995. Engendering Reproductive Policy and Practice in Peasant China: For a Feminist Demography of Reproduction. *Signs* 20 (3): 601–641.

Gu, Sujuan, Liuqu Zhuang, Yuhao Wu, and Feng Liu. 1994. Chinese IUDs. In *Proceedings from the Fourth International Conference on IUDs.* Edited by W. C. Bardin and D. R. Mishell. Newton, MA: Butterworth-Heinemann.

Gutiérrez, Elena R. 2008. *Fertile Matters: The Politics of Mexican-Origin Women's Reproduction.* Austin: University of Texas Press.

Guttmacher, Alan F. 1969. *Birth Control and Love: The Complete Guide to Contraception and Fertility*. 2nd ed. New York: Macmillan.

Haberland, Nicole, and Diana Measham, eds. 2002. *Responding to Cairo: Case Studies of Changing Practice in Reproductive Health and Family Planning*. New York: Population Council.

Halfon, Saul. 2000. Reconstructing Population Policy after Cairo: Demography, Women's Empowerment, and the Population Network. PhD diss., Cornell University.

Halfon, Saul. 2007. *The Cairo Consensus: Demographic Surveys, Women's Empowerment, and Regime Change in Population Policy*. Lanham, MD: Lexington Books.

Hall, Herbert H. 1962. The Stainless Steel Ring: An Effective and Safe Intra-Uterine Contraceptive Device. In *Intrauterine Contraceptive Devices: Proceedings of the First Conference on the IUCD (April 30–May 1962)*. Edited by C. Tietze and S. Lewit. New York: Excerpta Medica.

Haraway, Donna. 1988. Situated Knowledges: The Science Question in Feminism and the Privileged of Partial Perspective. *Feminist Studies* 14 (3): 575–599.

Haraway, Donna. 1991. Biopolitics of Postmodern Bodies: Determinations of Self in Immune System Discourse. In *Simians, Cyborgs, and Women: The Reinvention of Nature*. New York: Routledge.

Haraway, Donna. 1997. *Modest_Witness@Secone_Millenium.Femaleman_Meets_Oncomouse: Feminism and Technoscience*. New York: Routledge.

Haraway, Donna. 2000. *How Like a Leaf: An Interview with Thyrza Nichols Goodeve*. New York: Routledge.

Harding, Sandra. 1991. *Whose Science? Whose Knowledge? Thinking Women's Lives*. Ithaca, NY: Cornell University Press.

Harris, Colette. 2000. Control and Subversion: Gender, Islam, and Socialism in Tajikistan. PhD diss., University of Amsterdam.

Hartmann, Betsy. 1995. *Reproductive Rights and Wrongs: The Global Politics of Population Control*. Boston: South End Press.

Hawkins, Mary F. 1997. *Unshielded: The Human Cost of the Dalkon Shield*. Toronto: University of Toronto Press.

Hefnawi, Fouad, and Sheldon J. Segal, eds. 1975. *Analysis of Intrauterine Contraception: Proceedings of the Third International Conference on Intrauterine Contraception, Cairo, Arab Republic of Egypt, 12–14 December 1974*. Amsterdam: North-Holland.

Hicks, Karen M. 1994. *Surviving the Dalkon Shield IUD: Women Versus the Pharmaceutical Industry*. New York: Teachers College Press.

Hodgson, Dennis, and Susan Cotts Watkins. 1997. Feminists and Neo-Malthusians: Past and Present Alliances. *Population and Development Review* 23 (3): 469–523.

Hubacher, D., R. Lara-Ricalde, D. Taylor, F. Guerra-Infante, and R. Guzman-Rodriguez. 2001. Use of Copper Intrauterine Devices and the Risk of Tubal Infertility among Nulligravid Women. *New England Journal of Medicine* 345:561–567.

Huber, Sallie C., P. T. Piotrow, F. Barbara Orlans, and Geary Kommer. 1975. IUDs Reassessed: A Decade of Experience. *Population Reports,* Series B (2).

Indian Council of Medical Research. 1989. Randomized Clinical Trial with Intrauterine Devices: A 36-Month Study. *Contraception* 39 (1): 37–52.

International Planned Parenthood Federation. 1974. Republic of Korea (Family Planning). *IPPF Situation Report*:10.

Ishihama, Atsumi. 1959. Clinical Studies on Intrauterine Rings, Especially Present State of Contraception in Japan and the Experiences in the Use of Intrauterine Rings. *Yokohama Medical Journal* 10:89–105.

Jackson, Margaret. 1962. The Grafenberg Silver Ring in a Series of Patients Who Had Failed with Other Methods. In *Intrauterine Contraceptive Devices: Proceedings of the First Conference on the IUCD (April 30–May 1962).* Edited by C. Tietz and S. Lewit. New York: Excerpta Medica.

Jessen, Don. 1962. The Grafenberg Ring: A Clinical and Histopathologic Study. In *Intrauterine Contraceptive Devices: Proceedings of the First Conference on the IUCD (April 30–May 1962).* Edited by Christopher Tietz and Sarah Lewit. Amsterdam: Excerpta Medica.

Jones, Elise F., James R. Beniger, and Charles F. Westhoff. 1980. Pill and IUD Discontinuation in the United States, 1970–1975: The Influence of the Media. *Family Planning Perspectives* 12 (6): 293–300.

Joyce, Patrick. 2003. *The Rule of Freedom: Liberalism and the Modern City.* London: Verso.

Kamal, Ibrahim. 1979. *Atlas of Hysterographic Studies of the "IUD-Holding Uterus": Mode of Action and Evaluation of Side Effects of Intrauterine Contraception.* Ottawa, Canada: International Development Research Centre.

Kapsalis, Terri. 1997. *Public Privates: Performing Gynecology from Both Ends of the Speculum.* Durham, NC: Duke University Press.

Kaufman, David W., Jane Watson, Lynn Rosenberg, Susan P. Helmrich, Donald Miller, Olli S. Mietinen, Paul D. Stolley, and Samuel Shapiro. 1983. The Effect of Different Types of Intrauterine Devices on the Risk of Pelvic Inflammatory Disease. *Journal of the American Medical Association* 250 (6): 759–762.

Kennedy, T. G. 1997. Physiology of Implantation. Paper presented at the Tenth World Congress on In Vitro Fertilization and Assisted Reproduction, Vancouver, Canada, May 24–28.

Kim, Sonja. 2008. "Limiting Birth": Birth Control in Colonial Korea (1910–1945). *EASTS: East Asian Science and Technology Studies: An International Journal* 2 (3): 335–360.

Klitsch, Michael 1988. The Return of the IUD. *Family Planning Perspectives* 20 (1): 19, 40.

Koh, L. Y., and W. R. Jones. 1982. The Rosette Inhibition Test in Early Pregnancy Diagnosis. *Clinical Reproduction and Fertility* 1:229–233.

Krengel, Monika, and Katarian Greifeld. 2000. Uzbekistan in Transition: Changing Concepts in Family Planning and Reproductive Health. In *Contraception across Cultures: Technologies, Choices, Constraints.* Edited by A. Russell, E. J. Sobo, and M. Thompson. Oxford: Berg.

Kronmal, Richard, Coralyn W. Whitney, and Stephen D. Mumford. 1991. The Intrauterine Device and Pelvic Inflammatory Disease: The Women's Health Study Reanalyzed. *Journal of Clinical Epidemiology* 44:109–122.

Larimore, Walter L. 1999. Letter to the Editor: The Potential Postfertilization Effect with Use of the IUD. *American Family Physician* 60 (3): 761.

Latour, Bruno. 1987. *Science in Action: How to Follow Scientists and Engineers through Society.* Cambridge, MA: Harvard University Press.

Latour, Bruno. 1996. *Aramis, or the Love of Technology.* Cambridge, MA: Harvard University Press.

Latour, Bruno. 2003. Why Has Critique Run out of Steam? From Matters of Fact to Matters of Concern. *Critical Inquiry* 30:225–248.

Laveaga, Gabriela Soto. 2009. *Jungle Laboratories: Mexican Peasants, National Projects, and the Making of the Pill.* Durham, NC: Duke University Press.

Lee, Nancy C., George L. Rubin, and Robert Borucki. 1988. The Intrauterine Device and Pelvic Inflammatory Disease Revisited: New Results from the Women's Health Study. *Obstetrics and Gynecology* 72: 1–6.

Lee, Nancy C., Geirge L. Rubin, Howard W. Ory, and Ronald T. Burkman. 1983. Type of Intrauterine Device and the Risk of Pelvic Inflammatory Disease. *Obstetrics and Gynecology* 62:1–6.

Lehfeldt, Hans. 1962. Experience with Intrauterine Devices, 1928–1962. In *Intrauterine Contraceptive Devices: Proceedings of the First Conference on the IUCD (April 30- May 1962).* Edited by Christopher Tietz and Sarah Lewit. Amsterdam: Excerpta Medica.

Leonard, Eileen. 2003. *Women. Technology, and the Myth of Progress.*Upper Saddle River, NJ: Prentice-Hall.

Lindsay, Christina. 2003. From the Shadows: Users as Designers, Producers, Marketers, Distributors, and Technical Support. In *How Users Matter: The Co-Construction of*

Users and Technologies. Edited by Nelly Oudshoorn and Trevor Pinch. Cambridge, MA: MIT Press.

Lippes, Jack. 1962. A Study of Intra-Uterine Contraception: Development of a Plastic Loop. In *Intrauterine Contraceptive Devices: Proceedings of the First Conference on the IUCD (April 30–May 1962).* Edited by Christopher Tietze and Sarah Lewit. Amsterdam: Excerpta Medica.

Liskin, Laurie. 1982. IUDs: An Appropriate Contraceptive for Many Women. *Population Reports* Series B (4).

Loe, Meika. 2004. *The Rise of Viagra: How the Little Blue Pill Changed Sex in America.* New York: New York University Press.

Luukkainen, Tapani. 1994. Progestin-Releasing Intrauterine Contraceptive Device. In *Proceedings from the Fourth International Conference on IUDs.* Edited by C. W. Bardin and Daniel R. Mishell Jr. Boston: Butterworth-Heinemann.

Luukkainen, Tapani, and Juhani Toivonen. 1995. Levonorgestrel-Releasing IUD as a Method of Contraception with Therapeutic Properties. *Contraception* 52:269–276.

MacKenzie, Donald, and Judith Wajcman. 1999. *The Social Shaping of Technology.* Buckingham: Open University Press.

Mahadevan, Kuttan, Chi-Hsien Tuan, Jingyuan Yu, P. Krishnan, and M. Sumngala. 1994. *Differential Development and Demographic Dilemma.* Delhi: B. R. Publishing Co.

Mamo, Laura, and Jennifer Fishman. 2004. Potency in All the Right Places: Viagra as a Technology of the Gendered Body. *Body and Society* 7 (4): 13–35.

Mamo, Laura, and Jennifer Ruth Fosket. 2009. Scripting the Body: Pharmaceuticals and the (Re)Making of Menstruation. *Signs* 34 (4): 925–949.

Mann, Edwards C. 1962. Cineradiographic Observations on Intra-Uterine Contraceptive Devices. In *Intrauterine Contraceptive Devices: Proceedings of the First Conference on the IUCD (April 30–May 1962).* Edited by Christopher Tietz and Sarah Lewit. Amsterdam: Excerpta Medica.

Mann, Michael. 2003. Mapping the Country: European Geography and the Cartographical Construction of India, 1760–90. *Science, Technology and Society* 8 (1): 25–46.

Margulies, Lazar C. 1962. Permanent Reversible Contraception with an Intra-Uterine Plastic Spiral (Perma-Spiral). In *Intrauterine Contraceptive Devices: Proceedings of the First Conference on the IUCD (April 30–May 1962).* Edited by Christopher Tietz and Sarah Lewit. Amsterdam: Excerpta Medica.

Marks, Lara V. 2001. *Sexual Chemistry: A History of the Contraceptive Pill.* New Haven, CT: Yale University.

Martin, Emily. 2001. *The Woman in the Body: A Cultural Analysis of Reproduction*. Boston: Beacon Press.

Martin, Emily. 1991. The Egg and the Sperm: How Science Constructed a Romance Based on Stereotypical Male-Female Roles. *Signs* 16 (3): 485–501.

Mason, Carol. 2002. *Killing for Life: The Apocalyptic Narrative of Pro-Life Politics*. Ithaca, NY: Cornell University Press.

May, Elaine Tyler. 2010. *America and the Pill: A History of Promise, Peril, and Liberation*. New York: Basic Books.

McCann, Carole. 1994. *Birth Control Politics in the United States, 1916–1945*. Ithaca, NY: Cornell University Press.

McCann, Carole. 2009. Malthusian Men and Demographic Transitions: A Case Study of Hegemonic Masculinity in Mid-Twentieth Century Population Theory. *Frontiers: A Journal of Women's Studies* 30 (1): 142–171.

McCullough, Marie. 2010. IUD Usage Is on the Rise in U.S. *The Philadelphia Inquirer*, August 31, 2010.

Meldrum, Marcia L. 1996. "Simple Methods" and "Determined Contraceptors": The Statistical Evaluation of Fertility Control, 1957–1968. *Bulletin of the History of Medicine* 70 (2): 266–295.

Merchant, Carolyn. 1983. *The Death of Nature: Women, Ecology, and Scientific Revolution*. New York: HarperCollins.

Mintz, Morton. 1973. Doctors Attack IUD Safety. *Washington Post*, May 31.

Mintz, Morton. 1985. *At Any Cost: Corporate Greed, Women, and the Dalkon Shield*. New York: Pantheon Books.

Mishell, D. R., Jr. 1975a. Assessing the Intrauterine Device. *Family Planning Perspectives* 7:103–111.

Mishell, Daniel R. 1975b. IUD Revisited: Daniel R. Mishell, Jr. Replies. *Family Planning Perspectives* 7 (6): 246–247.

Mooney, Chris. 2005. *The Republican War on Science*. New York: Basic Books.

Moskowitz, Ellen H., and Bruce Jennings, eds. 1996. *Coerced Contraception? Moral and Policy Challenges of Long-Acting Birth Control*. Washington, DC: Georgetown University Press.

Moskowitz, Ellen H., Bruce Jennings, and Daniel Callahan. 1995. Long-Acting Contraceptives: Ethical Guidance for Policymakers and Health Care Providers. *Hastings Center Report* 25 (1): S1–S8.

Mumford, S., and E. Kessel. 1992. Was the Dalkon Shield a Safe and Effective IUD? The Conflict between Case-Control and Clinical Trial Study Findings. *Fertility and Sterility* 57:1151–1176.

Nathanson, Constance. 1991. *Dangerous Passage: The Social Construction of Sexuality in Women's Adolescence.* Philadelphia: Temple University Press.

Ong, Aihwa. 1995. Making the Biopolitical Subject: Cambodian Immigrants, Refugee Medicine, and Cultural Citizenship in California. *Social Science and Medicine* 40 (9): 1243–1257.

Onorato, Suzanne A. 1990. Organizational Legitimacy and the Social Construction of Contraceptives: The Politics of Technological Choice. PhD diss., Duke University.

Oppenheimer, W. 1959. Prevention of Pregnancy by the Grafenberg Ring Method. *American Journal of Obstetrics and Gynecology* 78:446–454.

Orlans, F. Barbara. 1973. Copper IUDs: Performance to Date. *Population Reports* Series B (1).

Ortega, Adruaba O., Ana Amuchstegui, and Marta Rivas. 1998. "Because They Were Born from Me": Negotiating Women's Rights in Mexico. In *Negotiating Reproductive Rights: Women's Perspectives across Countries and Cultures.* Edited by R. P. Petchesky and K. Judd. London: Zed Books.

Ortiz, María E., and Horacio B. Croxatto. 1987. The Mode of Action of IUDs. *Contraception* 36 (1): 37–53.

Ortiz, María E., and Horacio B. Croxatto. 2007. Copper-T Intrauterine Device and Levonorgestrel Intrauterine System: Biological Bases of Their Mechanism of Action. *Contraception* 75 (Supplement): 16–30.

Ory, Howard W. 1978. A Review of the Association between Intrauterine Devices and Acute Pelvic Inflammatory Diseases. *Journal of Reproductive Medicine* 20 (4): 200–204.

Oudshoorn, Nelly. 1994. *Beyond the Natural Body: An Archeology of Sex Hormones.* New York: Routledge.

Oudshoorn, Nelly. 1996. The Decline of the One-Size-Fits-All Paradigm, or How Reproductive Scientists Try to Cope with Postmodernity. In *Between Monsters, Goddesses, and Cyborgs: Feminist Confrontations with Science, Medicine, and Cyberspace.* Edited by Nina Lyke and Rosi Braidotti. London: Zed Books.

Oudshoorn, Nelly. 2000. Imagined Men: Representations of Masculinities in Discourses on Male Contraceptive Technology. In *Bodies of Technology: Women's Involvement with Reproductive Medicine.* Edited by A. R. Saetnan, Nelly Oudshoorn, and M. Kirejczyk. Columbus: Ohio State University.

Oudshoorn, Nelly. 2003a. Clinical Trials as a Cultural Niche in Which to Configure the Gender Identities of Users: The Case of Male Contraceptive Development. In *How Users Matter: The Co-Configuration of Users and Technologies*. Edited by Nelly Oudshoorn and Trevor Pinch. Cambridge, MA: MIT Press.

Oudshoorn, Nelly. 2003b. *The Male Pill: A Biography of a Technology in the Making.* Durham, NC: Duke University Press.

Oudshoorn, Nelly, and Trevor Pinch, eds. 2003. *How Users Matter: The Co-Construction of Users and Technologies*. Cambridge, MA: MIT Press.

Oudshoorn, Nelly, and Trevor Pinch. 2003. Introduction: How Users and Non-Users Matter. In *How Users Matter: The Co-Construction of Users and Technologies*. Edited by Nelly Oudshoorn and Trevor Pinch. Cambridge, MA: MIT Press.

Patrick, Joyce. 2003. *The Rule of Freedom: Liberalism and the Modern City.* London: Verso.

Perry, Susan L., and James L. Dawson. 1985. *Nightmare: Women and the Dalkon Shield.* New York: Macmillan .

Petchesky, Rosalind P. 1984. *Abortion and Woman's Choice.* New York: Longman.

Petchesky, Rosalind P., and Karen Judd, eds. 1998. *Negotiating Reproductive Rights: Women's Perspectives across Countries and Cultures.* London: Zed Books.

Piccinino, Linda J., and William D Mosher. 1998. Trends in Contraceptive Use in the United States: 1982–1995. *Family Planning Perspectives* 30 (1): 4–10, 46.

Pigg, Stacy Leigh. 2001. Languages of Sex and Aids in Nepal: Notes on the Social Production of Commensurability. *Cultural Anthropology* 16 (4): 481–541.

Pigg, Stacy Leigh. 2005. *Sex in Development: Science, Sexuality, and Morality in Global Perspective.* Durham, NC: Duke University Press.

Piotrow, Phyllis, Ward Rinehart, and John C. Schmidt. 1979. IUDs: Update on Safety, Effectiveness, and Research. *Population Reports* Series B (3).

Planned Parenthood Federation of Korea. 1973. Mother's Club of the Month. *PPFK Activity Report* 17:4.

Population Council. 1955. *Annual Report, 1952–55.* New York: Population Council.

Population Council. 1961. *Annual Report, 1961.* New York: Population Council.

Population Council. 1963. *Annual Report, 1963.* New York: Population Council.

Population Council. 1966. *Annual Report, 1966.* New York: Population Council.

Population Council. 1967. *Annual Report, 1967.* New York: Population Council.

Population Council. 1970. *Annual Report, 1970.* New York: Population Council.

Population Council. 1971. *Annual Report, 1971*. New York: Population Council.

Population Council. 1973. *Annual Report, 1973*. New York: Population Council.

Population Council. 1975. *Annual Report, 1975*. New York: Population Council.

Population Council. 1976. *Annual Report, 1976*. New York: Population Council.

Population Council. 1983. *Annual Report, 1983*. New York: Population Council.

Porter, Theodore M. 1992. Quantification and the Accounting Ideal in Science. *Social Studies of Science* 22:633–652.

Porter, Theodore M. 1995. *Trust in Numbers: The Pursuit of Objectivity in Science and Public Life*. Princeton, NJ: Princeton University Press.

Prager, Sarah, and Philip D. Darney. 2007. The Levonorgestrel Intrauterine System in Nulliparous Women. *Contraception* 75 (S): S12–S15.

Rabinow, Paul, and Nikolas Rose. 2006. "Biopower Today." *BioSocieties* 1 (2):195–217.

Rademacher, K., E. McGinn, R. Jacobstein, I. Yacobson, and V. Halpern. 2009. *Essential Knowledge About LNG-IUS (Mirena)*. Washington, DC: USAID. Downloaded from http://www.k4health.org/toolkits/iud/essential-knowledge-5 (accessed March 2011).

Ramirez de Arellano, A. B., and C. Seipp. 1983. *Colonialism, Catholicism, and Contraception: A History of Birth Control in Puerto Rico*. Chapel Hill: University of North Carolina Press.

Ramirez, Francisco J., and Ann M. Starrs. 1987. The Ending of IUD Sales in the United States: What Are the International Implications? *International Family Planning Perspectives* 13 (2): 71–74.

Rarick, Lisa. 2007. United States Regulatory Considerations for Intrauterine Progestin for Hormone Replacement Treatment. *Contraception* 75 (S6): S140–S143.

Rauh, Joseph L., and Robert L. Burket. 1975. The IUD Revisited. *Family Planning Perspectives* 7 (6): 244.

Razzak, Mohamed K. A. 1962. Intra-Uterine Contraceptive Devices. In *Intrauterine Contraceptive Devices: Proceedings of the First Conference on the IUCD (April 30–May 1962)*. Edited by Christopher Tietze and Sarah Lewit. Amsterdam: Excerpta Medica.

Reed, James. 1983. *The Birth Control Movement and American Society: From Private Vice to Public Virtue*. Princeton, NJ: Princeton University Press.

Reid, Frances. 1995. *Skin Deep*. Iris Films.

Riedmann, Agnes. 1993. *Science That Colonizes: A Critique of Fertility Studies in Africa*. Philadelphia: Temple University Press.

Rolfe, B. E. 1982. Detection of Fetal Wastage. *Fertility and Sterility* 37:655–660.

Rose, Nikolas, and Peter Miller. 1992. Political Power beyond the State: Problematics of Government. *British Journal of Sociology* 43 (2): 172–205.

Ruzek, Sheryl B. 1978. *The Women's Health Movement: Feminist Alternative to Medical Control.* New York: Praeger.

Salem, Ruwaida M. 2006. New Attention to the IUD. *Population Reports* Series B (7).

Sanders, Eli. 2000. $200 to Curb an Addict's Fertility: Controversial Programs Finds Willing Takers in Seattle. *Seattle Times*, April 13.

Sawicki, Jana. 1991. *Disciplining Foucault.* New York: Routledge.

Schiebinger, Londa. 2004. *Nature's Body: Gender in the Making of Modern Science.* New Brunswick, NJ: Rutgers University Press.

Schoen, Joanna. 2005. *Choice and Coercion: Birth Control, Sterilization, and Abortion in Public Health and Welfare.* Chapel Hill: University of North Carolina Press.

Scommegna, Antonio, Theresita Avila, Manuel Luna, and W. Paul Dmowski. 1974. Fertility Control by Intrauterine Release of Progesterone. *Obstetrics and Gynecology* 43 (5): 769–779.

Scommegna, Antonio, Geeta N. Pandya, Miriam Christ, Alice Lee, and Melvin R. Cohen. 1970. Intrauterine Administration of Progesterone by a Slow Releasing Device. *Fertility and Sterility* 21 (3): 201–210.

Scott, Roger B. 1968a. Critical Illness and Deaths Associated with Intrauterine Devices. *Obstetrics and Gynecology* 31:322.

Scott, Roger B. 1968b. *Report on Intrauterine Contraceptive Devices.* Washington, DC: FDA Advisory Committee on Obstetrics and Gynecology, Food and Drug Administration.

Seaman, Barbara. 1969. *The Doctor's Case against the Pill.* New York: P. H. Wyden.

Seaman, Barbara, and Gideon Seaman. 1977. *Women and the Crisis in Sex Hormones.* New York: Rawson Associates.

Segal, Sheldon J. 1997. Intrauterine Contraceptive Devices Act before Fertilization. *American Journal of Obstetrics and Gynecology* 177 (4): 980.

Segal, Sheldon. 2003. *Under the Banyan Tree: A Population Scientist's Odyssey.* New York: Oxford University Press.

Segal, Sheldon J., Francisco V. Alvarez, Christopher A. Adejuwon, Vivian Brache de Mejia, Patricia Leon, and Anibal Faundes. 1985. Absence of Chorionic Gonadotropin in Sera of Women Who Use Intrauterine Devices. *Fertility and Sterility* 44 (2): 214–218.

Segal, Sheldon J., Anna L. Southam, and K. D. Shafer, eds. 1965. *Intra-Uterine Contraception: Proceedings of the Second International Conference. October 2–3, 1964, New York City. Sponsored by the Population Council*. New York: Excerpta Medica Foundation.

Sen, Gita, Adrienne Germain, and Lincoln C. Chen, eds. 1994. *Population Policies Reconsidered: Health, Empowerment, and Rights*. New York: International Women's Health Coalition.

Silliman, Jael, Marlene Gerber Fried, Loretta Ross, and Elena R. Gutierrez, eds. 2004. *Undivided Rights: Women of Color Organize for Reproductive Justice*. Boston: South End Press.

Sivin, Irvin 1989. IUDs Are Contraceptives, Not Abortifacients: A Comment on Research and Belief. *Studies in Family Planning* 20:355–359.

Sivin, Irvin 1993. Another Look at the Dalkon Shield: Meta-Analysis Underscores Its Problems. *Contraception* 48:1–12, 192.

Sivin, Irvin, Janet Stern, Elsimar Coutinho, Carlos Mattos, Sayed El Mahgoub, Soledad Diaz, Margarita Pavez, et al. 1991. Prolonged Intrauterine Contraception: A Seven-Year Randomized Study of Levonorgestrel 20mcg/Day (Lng 20) and Copper T380 Ag IUDs. *Contraception* 44 (5): 473–480.

Smart, Y. C., L. S. Fraser, and T. K. Roberts. 1983. Fertilization and Early Pregnancy Loss in Healthy Women Attempting Contraception. *Clinical Reproduction and Fertility* 1 (3):177–184.

Smith, Andrea. 2005a. Beyond Pro-Choice Versus Pro-Life: Women of Color and Reproductive Justice. *NWSA Journal* 17 (1): 119–140.

Smith, Andrea. 2005b. *Conquest: Sexual Violence and American Indian Genocide*. Boston: South End Press.

Sobol, R. B. 1991. *Bending the Law: The Story of the Dalkon Shield Bankruptcy*. Chicago: University of Chicago Press.

Spinnato, Joseph A. 1997. Mechanism of Action of Intrauterine Contraceptive Devices and Its Relation to Informed Consent. *American Journal of Obstetrics and Gynecology* 176:503–506.

Stanford, J. B., and R. T. Mikolajczyk. 2002. Mechanisms of Action of Intrauterine Devices: Update and Estimation of Postfertilization Effects. *American Journal of Obstetrics and Gynecology* 187 (6): 1699–1708.

Stangel, Rebecca. 2009. Plan B and the Doctrine of Double Effect: It's Not Like Abortion, Even If It Sometimes Ends Pregnancy. *Hastings Center* 39 (4): 21–25.

Stanwood, Nancy L., Joanne M. Garrett, and Thomas R. Konrad. 2002. Obstetrician-Gynecologists and the Intrauterine Device: A Survey of Attitudes and Practice. *Obstetrics and Gynecology* 99:275–280.

Stark, Nancy. 2000. My Body, My Problem: Contraceptive Decision-Making among Rural Bangladeshi Women. In *Contraception across Cultures: Technologies, Choices, Constraints.* Edited by A. Russell, E. J. Sobo, and M. Thompson. Oxford: Berg.

Stoler, A. L., C. McGranahan, and P. C. Perdue, eds. 2008. *Imperial Formations.* Santa Fe, NM: School for Advanced Research Press.

Szaller, Jim. 1999. One Lawyer's 25 Year Journey: The Dalkon Shield Saga. *Ohio Trial* 9 (4): 7–20.

Takeshita, Chikako. 2004. Contraceptive Technology and Reproductive Rights: The IUD at Historical and Geographical Junctures. *Advances in Gender Research* 8:251–284.

Takeshita, Chikako. 2010. The IUD in Me: On Embodying Feminist Technoscience Studies. *Science as Culture* 19(1): 37–60.

Tandon, Aditi. 2010. Health Innovations: Two Indian Scientists Get Bill Gates's Grant. *Tribune* (Chandigarh, India), Nov. 10. http://www.tribuneindia.com/2010/20101110/main5.htm (accessed March 2011).

Tatum, Howard J. 1975. Morphological Studies of Dalkon Shield Tails Removed from Patients. *Contraception* 11 (4): 465–477.

Tatum, Howard J. 1976. Transport of Bacteria by the Dalkon Shield. *Journal of the American Medical Association* 235 (7): 704–705.

Tatum, Howard J., Frederick Schmidt, David Phillips, Maclyn McCarty, and William M. O'Leary. 1975. The Dalkon Shield Controversy: Structural and Bacteriological Studies of IUD Tails. *Journal of the American Medical Association* 231 (7): 711–717.

Thompson, Mary S. 2000. Family Planning or Reproductive Health? Interpreting Policy and Providing Family Planning Services in Highland Chiapas, Mexico. In *Contraceptives across Culture: Technologies, Choices, Constraints.* Edited by A. Russell, E. J. Sobo, and M. S. Thompson. Oxford: Berg.

Tietze, Christopher. 1962. Intra-Uterine Contraceptive Rings: History and Statistical Appraisal. In *Intrauterine Contraceptive Devices: Proceedings of the First Conference on the IUCD (April 30–May 1962).* Edited by Christopher Tietze and Sarah Lewit. New York: Excerpta Medica.

Tietze, Christopher. 1968. Intrauterine Contraception: A Research Report. *Studies in Family Planning* 36:11–12.

Tietze, Christopher. 1969. Modern Methods of Birth Control. In *Family Planning Programs: An International Survey.* Edited by Bernard Berelson. New York: Basic Books.

Tietze, Christopher, and Sarah Lewit, eds. 1962. *Intrauterine Contraceptive Devices: Proceedings of the First Conference on the IUCD (April 30- May 1962).* Amsterdam, London, New York: Excerpta Medica.

Tietze, Christopher, and Sarah Lewit eds. 1968. Clinical Experience with Intra-Uterine Devices: Pregnancies, Expulsions, and Removals. *Journal of Reproduction and Fertility* 17:443–457.

Tietze, Christopher, and Sarah Lewit eds. 1970. Evaluation of the Intrauterine Device: Ninth Progress Report of the Cooperative Statistical Program. *Studies in Family Planning* 55:1–40.

Tone, Andrea. 1997. *Controlling Reproduction: An American History*. Wilmington: SR Books.

Tone, Andrea. 1999. Violence by Design: Contraceptive Technology and the Invasion of the Female Body. In *Lethal Imagination: Violence and Brutality in American History*. Edited by Michael A. Bellesiles. New York: New York University Press.

Tone, Andrea. 2001. *Devices and Desires: A History of Contraceptives in America*. New York: Hill and Wang.

Toulemon, Laurent, and Henri Leridon. 1998. Contraceptive Practices and Trends in France. *Family Planning Perspectives* 30 (3):114–120.

Treiman, Katherine, and Laurie Liskin. 1988. IUDs: A New Look. *Population Reports* Series B (5).

Treiman, Katherine, Laurie Liskin, Adriennne Kols, and Ward Rinehart. 1995. IUDs: An Update. *Population Reports* Series B (6).

Trussell, James, A. M. Lalla, and Q. V. Doan. 2008. Cost-Effectiveness Analysis of Contraceptives Available in the United States. *Contraception* 78 (2): 177–178.

United Nations. 1995. *Report of the International Conference on Population and Development*. Cairo: United Nations.

van Kammen, Jessika. 2000. Do Users Matter? In *Bodies of Technology: Women's Involvement with Reproductive Medicine*. Edited by A. R. Saetnan, Nelly Oudshoorn, and M. Kirejczyk. Columbus: Ohio State University.

van Kammen, Jessika, and Nelly Oudshoorn. 2002. Gender and Risk Assessment in Contraceptive Technologies. *Sociology of Health and Illness* 24 (4): 436–461.

Warwick, Anderson. 2006. *Colonial Pathologies: Hygiene, Race, and Science in the Philippines*. Durham, NC: Duke University Press.

Watkins, Elizabeth. 1998. *On the Pill: A Social History of Oral Contraceptives, 1950–1970*. Baltimore: Johns Hopkins University Press.

Watkins, Elizabeth Siegel. 2010a. From Breakthrough to Bust: The Brief Life of Norplant, the Contraceptive Implant. *Journal of Women's History* 22 (3): 88–111.

Watkins, Elizabeth Siegel. 2010b. The Social Construction of a Contraceptive Technology: An Investigation of the Meaning of Norplant. *Science, Technology, and Human Values* 36 (1): 33–54.

Weilerstein, Ralph W. 1957. The Hazards of Intrauterine Pessaries: An Evaluation. *Western Journal of Surgery, Obstetrics, and Gynecology* 65(3): 157–160.

Westoff, Charles F. 1972. The Modernization of U.S. Contraceptive Practice. *Family Planning Perspectives* 4:10–12.

Whelan, Elizabeth M. 1975. Attitudes toward Menstruation. *Studies in Family Planning* 6 (4): 106–108.

WHO. 1981. A Cross-Cultural Study of Menstruation: Implications for Contraceptive Development and Use. *Studies in Family Planning* 12 (1): 3–16.

WHO. 1996. *Improving Access to Quality Care in Family Planning: Medical Eligibility Criteria for Initiating and Continuing Use of Contraceptive Methods*. Geneva: WHO.

Whyte, Susan Reynolds, Sjaak van der Geest, and Anita Hardon. 2002. *Social Lives of Medicines*. Cambridge: Cambridge University Press.

Wilcox, Allen J., Donna Day Baird, and Clarice R. Weinberg. 1999. Time of Implantation of the Conceptus and Loss of Pregnancy. *New England Journal of Medicine* 340 (23): 1796–1799.

Wilcox, Allen J., Clarice R. Weinberg, E. Glenn Armstrong, and Robert E. Canfield. 1987. Urinary Human Chorionic Gonadotropin among Intrauterine Device Users: Detection with a Highly Specific and Sensitive Assay. *Fertility and Sterility* 47:265–269.

Winner, Langdon. 1986. Do Artifacts Have Politics? In *The Whale and the Reactor: A Search for Limits in an Age of High Technology*. Chicago: University of Chicago Press.

Wood, Clive. 1971. *Intrauterine Devices*. London: Butterworth.

Woolgar, Steve. 1991. Configuring the User: The Case of Usability Trials. In *A Sociology of Monsters: Essays on Power, Technology, and Domination*. Edited by John Law. New York: Routledge.

Zipper, J. 1969. Suppression of Fertility by Intrauterine Copper and Zinc in Rabbits. A New Approach to Intrauterine Contraception. *American Journal of Obstetrics and Gynecology* 105:529–534.

Index

Italicized page numbers indicate illustrations.

Printed in the United States
by Baker & Taylor Publisher Services